Deborah Mills   Carole Fraser

THERAPEUTIC ACTIVITIES FOR THE UPPER LIMB

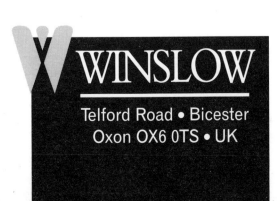

WINSLOW

Telford Road • Bicester
Oxon OX6 0TS • UK

First published in 1989 by
Winslow Press Limited, Telford Road, Bicester, Oxon
OX6 0TS
Reprinted 1990, 1991, 1992, 1994, 1995

Illustrations by Gabrielle Nunn

Phototypset by Gecko Limited, Bicester, Oxon

02–282 Printed in Great Britain (HtP)

British Library Cataloguing in Publication Data
Mills, Deborah
    Therapeutic activities for the upper limb.
    1. Man. Limbs. Injuries. Therapy
    I. Title   II. Fraser, Carole
    617'.58004
    ISBN 0–86388–059–2

Contents

List of Activities ■ v

List of Abbreviations ■ vi

Acknowledgements ■ vi

Introduction ■ 1

How to Use this Manual ■ 2

Purposeful Activity & Therapeutic
Exercise in the Context of OT ■ 5

Movements ■ 7

Use of Computer Switches ■ 137

Index ■ 147

Deborah Mills

DEBORAH MILLS received a Bachelor of Science degree in Rehabilitation Medicine (Occupational Therapy and Physiotherapy) from the University of British Columbia in 1979. She worked in paediatrics until 1984, first as a physiotherapist and later as an occupational therapist in several Canadian schools and hospitals. In the following two years, she was an occupational therapist and micro-computer program co-ordinator at a regional spinal cord rehabilitation centre, Lyndhurst Hospital in Toronto, Ontario.

During 1986–87 she worked closely with Carole Fraser in the OT department at Addenbrooke's Hospital, Cambridge. Currently practising as a Senior Occupational Therapist in the areas of specialised seating, computers and technical aids for the disabled, she is now based at the Greater Victoria Hospital Society in Victoria, British Columbia.

Carole Fraser

CAROLE FRASER trained at Dorset House School of Occupational Therapy in Oxford. She gained a BA (Hons) degree from the Open University in 1987 and was also awarded a Churchill Travel Fellowship in the same year to study prosthetics in America and Canada.

After qualifying as an occupational therapist she worked in orthopaedic, geriatric and acute physical hospitals and also taught at St Loyes School of Occupational Therapy at Exeter.

Currently Head Occupational Therapist in the Acute Unit at Addenbrooke's Hospital, Cambridge, her particular clinical and research interests are motor control and acquisition and retraining of motor skills.

List of Activities

Bandage Roll/90
Beads/118
Braintease/44
Bricks/32

Chopping/40
Clothes-Peg Sheep/131
Coin Travel/106
Computer Switch Elevation/Depression/145
Computer Switch Protraction/Retraction/138
Computerised FEPS/141

Darts/80
Dowel: pronation/supination/68
Dowel: shoulder abduction/adduction/48
Dowel: shoulder horizontal abduction/
        adduction/24
Dowel: shoulder rotation/54

Elastics/120

Finger Extension Game/93
Finger Ladder/46
Fluid Pump/127

Guillotining/37

Interossei Box/108
Interossei Sheep/110

Kneading/10
Knights/62

Lumbrical Box Game/95
Lumbrical Sanding/97

Magic Squares/20
Maze Game/12
Mercury Switch with Computer/143

Nuts and Bolts/116

Pin Solitaire/125
Ping Pong Puff/129
Post Box/82
Putty Pancake/123
Putty Pinch/133
Pyramids/50

Rolling Pastry/16

Sanding/34
Sheep/74
Shove Board/64
Skateboard/26
Ski Jump/84
Sponge Ball Squeeze/99
Spot Board/28
Stacking Bricks/32
Stick Printing/56
Suspended Ball Activity/59

Table Football/77
Threaded Solitaire I/72
Threaded Solitaire II/86
Tong Solitaire/103
T-Shape Solitaire/101
Tug O'War I/18
Tug O'War II/112
Tweezer Bead Art/135

Wire Maze/70

List of Abbreviations and Symbols

DIP   Distal interphalangeal
EMG   Electromyography
ER   External rotation
FEPs Flexion extension pronation supination
IP   Interphalangeal
IR   Internal rotation
MCP   Metacarpophalangeal
ROM   Range of movement
PIP   Proximal interphalangeal
~   At least

Acknowledgements

The authors would like to thank the following:

The OT Department, Addenbrooke's Hospital, Cambridge, United Kingdom

Steve Smart, BSc, MSc, Research Assistant, The Microcomputer Centre, The University of Dundee, United Kingdom

Alison Monteith, Toni Fine, Linda Collins, and OT staff, Royal National Orthopaedic Hospital, Stanmore, United Kingdom

Carole Roberts, Oddstock Hospital, Salisbury, United Kingdom

June Sutherland, Westminster Hospital, London

Christie Brenchley and Cathy Atkinson, Lyndhurst Hospital, Toronto, Ontario, Canada

Donna Martin, Orthopaedic and Arthritic Hospital, Toronto, Ontario, Canada

Sue Rugg, The London Hospital, London.

Doreen Rowland and the OT staff, Wolfson Medical Rehabilitation Centre, London.

Chris Mitchell and OT staff, Dundee Royal Infirmary, United Kingdom

. . . whose knowledge and experience assisted us in the development of this manual.

INTRODUCTION

The aim of this manual is to give guidelines for and examples of the use of therapeutic activities in treatment of the upper limb. The specific activities included here do not form an exhaustive list; each one indicates a role that it, and other activities similar to it, can play in a programme of treatment. These indicative activities are presented in a format that encourages occupational therapists to be analytical in their approach to the use of these or other activities in treatment.

The therapist may use the manual as an educational tool to indicate to the patient the purpose of the activity being used. The activities have been devised for treatment with adults, although some activities may be appropriate for use with children. While most of the equipment may already be in use in therapy departments, these activities provide innovative ways to adapt or use this equipment. This manual has been written for qualified occupational therapists: it assumes their professional discretion in the application of such activities to whatever treatment they undertake.

This manual falls into two sections, which contain:

▶ Some general theory on the use of therapeutic activities in the practice of occupational therapy; a description of how this manual can be most effectively used; definitions of the terminology used throughout.

▶ Individual activities for each movement of the upper limb, including:

a) diagrams of the muscles used for each movement;

b) the nerve supply and normal range of movement expected;

c) a task analysis of each activity, with extensive use of illustrations.

These therapeutic activities should only be used once a full assessment has been completed and problems and treatment goals identified. The therapist must be aware of limitations of the patient and contra-indications of treatment (*eg* increased tone, pain, decreased cognitive functioning, altered sensation) and take those into account before applying any of the activities.

The activities included in this manual can, for the most part, be carried out with equipment that:

a) is available in most therapy departments,
b) can be constructed easily and inexpensively, or
c) is commercially available.

Material on the use of computers as a motivator in the treatment of upper limbs is included to give insight as to what is currently available and where some of the future potential lies in this area.

It is hoped that this manual will be a stimulus for many innovative ideas. It does not profess to include all possible activities for treatment of the upper limb, rather to encourage a more analytical approach to the use of activities in therapy and to facilitate further ideas.

HOW TO USE THIS MANUAL

This manual can be used as a quick reference when designing or redesigning a treatment programme. It is important to complete an assessment of the patient to determine that therapeutic activities or exercises are an appropriate treatment modality and then which specific activities will best assist in the achievement of the stated treatment goals. To start, check the index to find the movement or movements that you want. Turn to the activities for that movement, read through the analysis, and decide which one or ones may help achieve the goals. For quick reference they have been categorised both as therapeutic activity or exercise, and as light or moderate, as defined below. Once an activity is selected it may then be appropriate to show the anatomical diagrams and activity information to the patient to help them better understand the purpose of the activity.

Terminology

The following terminology has been used within this manual:

Concentric (Isotonic) Contraction

During a concentric contraction there is joint motion and the muscle shortens. This can be done with or without resistance. Concentric contractions may be performed in positions with gravity assisting or gravity eliminated or against gravity, according to the clients muscle grade and the goal of the exercise *(Pedretti, LW, 1985, p132)*. An example of a concentric contraction of the biceps is lifting a bucket of sand up from the ground.

Eccentric Contraction

When muscles contract eccentrically, the tension in the muscle increases or remains constant while the muscle lengthens. This may be done with or without resistance. An example of an eccentric contraction performed against no resistance is the slow lowering of the arm to the table. The biceps are contracting eccentrically in this instance. An example of eccentric contraction against resistance is the controlled return of a bucket of sand lifted from the ground. Here, the biceps are contracting eccentrically to control the rate and co-ordination of the elbow extension in setting the bucket on the ground *(Pedretti, p132)*.

Isometric Contraction

During an isometric contraction there is no joint motion, and the muscle length remains the same. A muscle and its antagonist may be contracted at any point in the ROM to stabilise a joint. This may be without resistance or against some outside resistance, such as the therapist's hand or a table-top *(Pedretti, p132)*. An example of isometric exercise of biceps against resistance is pressing up underneath a table with the forearm in supination.

Concentric/Eccentric (vice versa)

When a movement is in one direction, one set of muscles may be using a concentric contraction and the opposite group of muscles may be using an eccentric contraction. However, when the movement is done in the opposite direction the opposition contractions may be used. In such cases, this has been indicated by 'conc/ecc (vv)'.

Fine Motor

For this manual, fine motor activity involves any hand function, either for stabilisation or active control.

Gross Motor

For this manual, gross motor includes any activity, either stabilisation or active movement, in the upper limb except the hand.

Muscle Grading System

Grade	Definition
0	No muscle contraction
1	Contraction can be felt, but there is no motion
2−	Part moves through an incomplete ROM with gravity eliminated
2	Part moves through a complete ROM with gravity eliminated
2+	Part moves through incomplete ROM (less than 50%) against gravity or through complete ROM with gravity eliminated against slight resistance
3−	Part moves through an incomplete ROM (more than 50%) against gravity
3	Part moves through complete ROM against gravity
3+	Part moves through a complete ROM against gravity and slight resistance
4	Part moves through a complete ROM against gravity and moderate resistance
5	Part moves through complete ROM against gravity and full resistance

(after Pedretti 1985)

Muscle Strength Categorisation

Light: Any activity requiring minimal resistance of Grade 3+ or less.
Moderate: Any activity requiring minimal resistance of more than Grade 3+.

Range of Motion

Range of motion (ROM) is described in terms of a portion of the normal range of the joint movement. For example, if the activity requires a minimum of approximately one half of shoulder flexion, and that range is required to be within the mid-range, it would be indicated as follows ~ ½ mid-range. At other times it may be described as the approximate minimum number of degrees of range required to complete that activity.

Purposeful Activity

Any activity which has an inherent goal other than the rehabilitation value.

Therapeutic Exercise

Any activity in which the only goal is the rehabilitation goal; it has no inherent goal within the activity itself.

Flow chart illustrating the therapy process

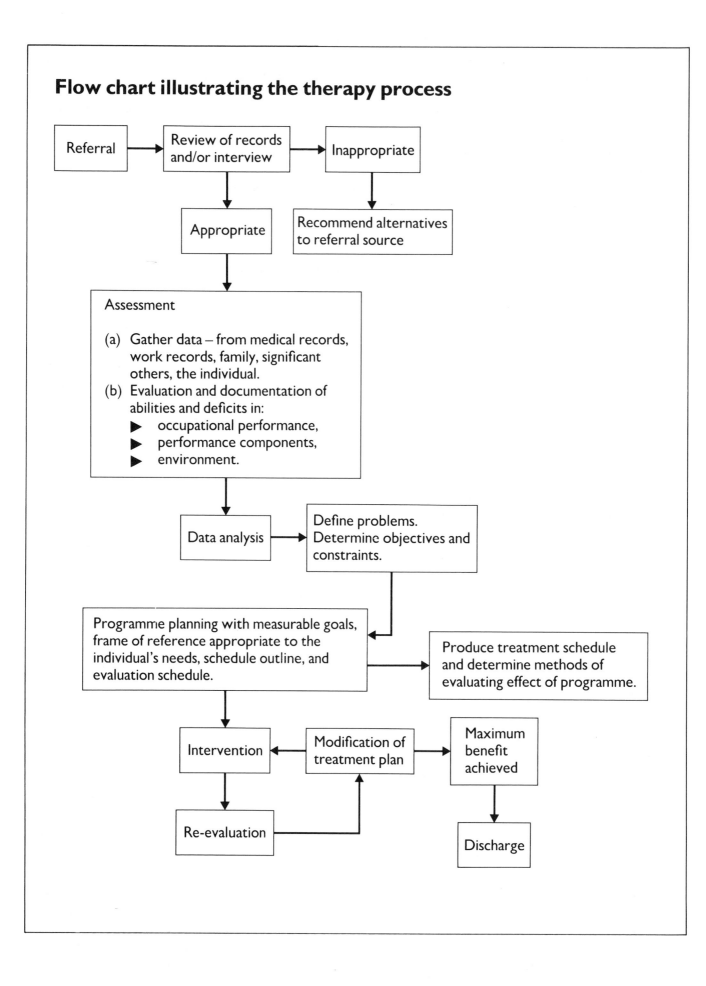

PURPOSEFUL ACTIVITY & THERAPEUTIC EXERCISE IN THE CONTEXT OF THERAPY

The terms 'purposeful activity' and 'therapeutic exercise' require clarification in the context of this manual.

Purposeful activity is a task in which individuals actively participate with their focus on the task itself rather than the exercise within it. For example, an individual participating in sanding a piece of wood may focus on the task of smoothing the wood rather than achieving the required movements of shoulder and elbow.

Therapeutic exercise directs the individual's attention to increasing a specific function such as strength or range of motion. There is no inherent goal within the activity itself. For example, a weight programme designed for strengthening muscles would be considered a therapeutic exercise.

A third term, 'therapeutic activity', covers both therapeutic exercise and purposeful activity and refers to any activity adapted by the therapist to achieve a therapeutic goal.

Occupational therapy has traditionally relied on the use of purposeful activity rather than therapeutic exercise and a departure from this is often seen as a threat to the profession. However 'purposeful activity' used to the exclusion of more specific techniques can give rise to some significant problems. The end product of a given task may become the principal motivation for performing the task. That in itself may appear beneficial as it encourages the patient to move the focus of attention away from the problem, but the patient may lose sight of the specific rehabilitation goal and use compensatory or incorrect movements which will not work effectively or efficiently in achieving the therapeutic goal. Too much time could be focused on how to produce a satisfactory end project or win a game when more efficient rehabilitation would be achieved by focusing the attention on perfecting motor control of a specific body part. When using a purposeful activity it is not always possible to achieve control in grading resistance, range of motion and repetition of specific movements. In the early stages of rehabilitation pure movement is often the most effective treatment and is best understood and accepted by the patient. Concentration on the pure movement is needed to fully utilize sensory feedback and monitor results in order to achieve a goal.

The authors consider both therapeutic exercise and purposeful activity important in achieving therapeutic goals. Both have been included in this manual to categorize the activities.

Methodology

Thorough assessment of individual patients is mandatory prior to choosing an activity which might be a therapeutic exercise or a purposeful activity. Rehabilitation goals must be clearly established and explained. The therapist must then ensure that the chosen activity meets those goals and is being correctly performed by the patient. Not only must the activity meet the physical goals but it must also be motivating in some way. Thorough and ongoing assessment will help the patient and therapist understand performance effectiveness. See the flow chart which illustrates the referral, assessment and reassessment process in occupational therapy.

In each activity positioning is vital in order to achieve the desired movement. Also, through alteration of position either of the activity or patient, other movements may be achieved. It is important to carefully observe the patient performing the activity to ensure that they are not using compensatory or trick movements to achieve the task. The activities used are usually against gravity. However, with creative positioning a gravity-eliminated position may be achieved. For example, for shoulder flexion, the patient could lie in a prone position on a plinth with their head over the end. The activity can then be performed on the floor beneath them.

Many adaptations can be incorporated into any activity. For those without active hand function many of the activities can be adapted with a cuff in which to place their hand. For those with weak grasp, a handle or game piece can often be built up.

It is important when choosing an activity that it is not too complex for the individual so that they lose sight of their goal. Often activities that are most effective are short in duration and use repetitive movements. It is very important that the patient understand the goal of the exercise and demonstrate some motivation to complete it.

Also we must always be careful of overuse of an activity – we often find an activity that achieves our end goal and use it to the exclusion of all else. Remember to be creative – there are always many ways of achieving one movement.

A treatment session may end with the incorporation of that movement into a simple functional activity which gives even more meaning to the treatment session.

Reasons for the Format

The task analysis that was developed for the purposes of this manual is only one method of breaking down activity. It has incorporated motor components alone, and has not considered the perceptual, cognitive, sensory, psychological or social components. It is intended only as a start to encourage therapists to be more analytical in their approach to the use of activities. In future, more in-depth analysis using scientific measurement tools may be used and many more activities analysed.

Movements

Shoulder Depression/Elevation ■ 9

Shoulder Protraction/Retraction ■ 15

Shoulder Horizontal Abduction/Adduction ■ 23

Shoulder Extension/Flexion ■ 31

Shoulder Abduction/Adduction ■ 43

Shoulder (Internal/External) Rotation ■ 53

Elbow Flexion/Extension ■ 61

Forearm Pronation/Supination ■ 67

Wrist Flexion/Extension ■ 79

MCP Flexion/Extension ■ 89

Finger Abduction/Adduction ■ 105

IP Flexion/Extension ■ 115

Grasp Strengthening ■ 127

Pinch Strengthening ■ 131

MOVEMENT

Shoulder Depression

Prime Movers

Trapezius (inferior fibres)

Normal Range

see diagram.

Range of Motion

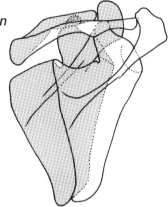

Nerve Supply

Spinal Accessory and branches from ($C_{3,4}$)

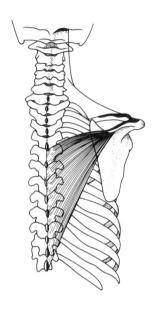

Trapezius (inferior fibres)

MOVEMENT

Shoulder Elevation

Prime Movers

Trapezius (superior fibres)

Levator Scapulae

Normal Range

see diagram.

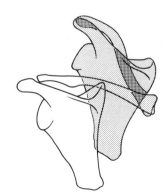

Nerve Supply

Spinal Accessory and branches from ($C_{3,4}$)

($C_{3,4}$) and frequently branch from dorsal scapular

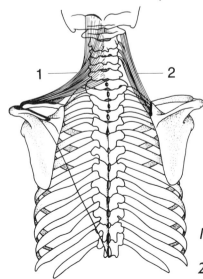

1 Trapezius (superior fibres)

2 Levator scapulae

TITLE

Kneading

MOVEMENT

Shoulder Depression/ Elevation

Category

Therapeutic Exercise, Light

Equipment

▶ adjustable height table;

▶ doughs or putty of varying consistency.

Description

Patient stands at adjustable height table set at hip level, dough is set out in front of them. With straight arms, knead the dough by pushing down through heel of hand, pushing action comes from shoulder depression. Lift up with shoulder elevation and repeat.

Skills required for activity as exercise
Action

Joints Used	Minimum Jt Range	Main Muscle Groups	Type of Contraction	Minimum Ms Grade
ACTIVE shoulder	full depression/ elevation	depressors elevators	conc/ecc. ecc/conc.	3+ 3+
STATIC elbows – fully extended wrists – fully extended hands – open				

Co-ordination

Gross Motor ■ control at shoulders; bilateral activity, both arms acting simultaneously.

Fine Motor ■ sustained open hand.

Gradation

	yes/no	How?
RESISTANCE	yes	alter stiffness or thickness of dough; can use theraputty or varying resistance.
RANGE OF MOTION	yes	alter table height.
CO-ORDINATION (gross/fine)	no	

Also used for:	How?
elbow flex/ext.	knead dough using elbow flexion and extension.

Comments

This can be incorporated into a functional activity if appropriate.

TITLE

Maze Game

MOVEMENT

Shoulder Depression

Category

Purposeful Activity, Light

Description

Patient sits at adjustable height table, with maze game at elbow level. Rest forearms in mid-position on platforms on game, elbows are flexed to about 90°. Start ball at outside of maze and by using a downward motion at one shoulder (shoulder depression) start to move the ball through maze, ending up with it in the centre. This can also be done standing with palms resting on platforms; keep elbows straight, and push down from shoulder.

Equipment

▶ wooden maze board with forearm platforms on each side; board is placed on a round bottomed surface (*see Figure 1*);

▶ adjustable height table.

Skills required for activity as exercise
Action

Joints Used	Minimum Jt Range	Main Muscle Groups	Type of Contraction	Minimum Ms Grade
ACTIVE shoulder	full depression	depressors	concentric	3+
STATIC shoulders – slightly flexed elbows – flexed to 90°				

Co-ordination

Gross Motor ■ control at shoulder;

■ co-ordination between left and right, one shoulder depressing and the other elevating.

Fine Motor ■ none.

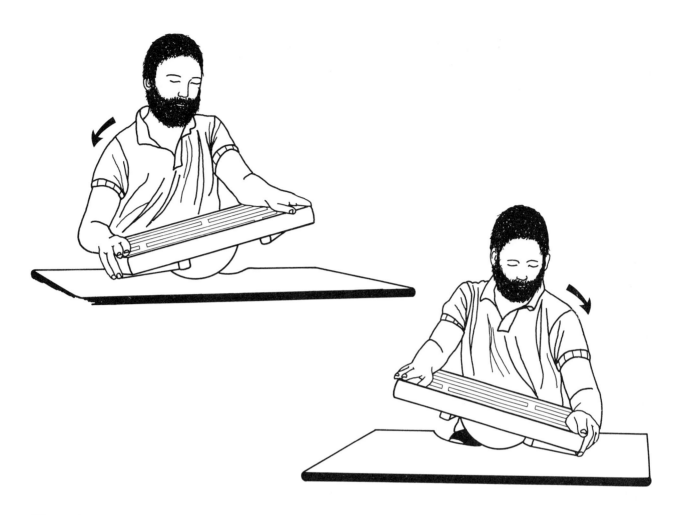

Figure 1

Gradation

	yes/no	How?
RESISTANCE	no	
RANGE OF MOTION	no	
CO-ORDINATION (gross/fine)	yes	alter size and complexity of maze

MOVEMENT

Shoulder Protraction

Prime Movers

Serratus Anterior

Nerve Supply

Long Thoracic ($C_{5,6,7}$)

MOVEMENT

Shoulder Retraction

Prime Movers

Rhomboid Major

Rhomboid Minor

Trapezius (middle fibres)

Nerve Supply

Dorsal Scapular (C_5)

Dorsal Scapular (C_5)

Spinal Accessory and branches from ($C_{3,4}$)

TITLE
Rolling Pastry

MOVEMENT
Shoulder Protraction/Retraction

Category

Therapeutic Exercise, Light

Description

Patient sits at adjustable height table, set at chest height. Place open hands, palm down at either end of rolling implement, starting with finger tips only on top. Roll forward, keeping elbows straight, thrusting forward from shoulders. Once as far forward as possible, without moving trunk forward, roll back to starting position. Can be done on bare table or with dough of varying thickness.

Equipment

▶ rolling pin or cylinder;

▶ adjustable height table;

▶ pastry or play dough if appropriate.

Skills required for activity as exercise
Action

Joints Used	Minimum Jt Range	Main Muscle Groups	Type of Contraction	Minimum Ms Grade
ACTIVE shoulder hand	a few degrees protr/retr. full ext.	protractors retractors extensors	conc/ecc. ecc/conc. concentric	2 2 3
STATIC shoulder at ~90° flex. elbow – fully extended wrist				

Co-ordination

Gross Motor ■ control at shoulder, co-ordination between protractors and retractors;

■ control of two arms working in the same action simultaneously.

Fine Motor ■ sustained open hand.

Gradation

	yes/no	How?
RESISTANCE	yes	do with or without dough; alter thickness of dough; roll up an inclined board.
RANGE OF MOTION	yes	can work within available range, starting with only a few degrees.
CO-ORDINATION (gross/fine)	no	

Also used for:	How?
1 shoulder flex/ext. 2 elbow ext/flex.	do up a steep incline using shoulder flex/ext. to roll. start with roller close to body, push out by straightening elbows and pull back by bending them.

Comments

The extent of ROM is only a few degrees, therefore the therapist must monitor closely, particularly for compensation with the trunk.

This can be incorporated into a functional kitchen activity if appropriate.

TITLE

Tug O' War I

MOVEMENT

Shoulder Protraction/Retraction

Category

Purposeful Activity, Light

Description

Patient stands or sits in front of rope that is attached to the wall at about chest height. Grasp rope with gross grasp, with straight arms. It may be necessary to stabilise patient's position with chest strap. Walk hand over hand forwards and backwards along the rope. Forward action is achieved with shoulder protraction and backwards action with shoulder retraction. Watch that patient is not compensating with forward and backward trunk movement (although some is to be expected).

Equipment

▶ thick rope or bath towel securely attached to wall, height should be adjustable.

Skills required for activity as exercise
Action

Joints Used	Minimum Jt Range	Main Muscle Groups	Type of Contraction	Minimum Ms Grade
ACTIVE shoulders	a few degrees protr/retr.	protractors retractors	conc/ecc. (vv) ecc/conc. (vv)	3+
hands	gross grasp partial opening	flexors extensors	concentric concentric	3+ 3−
STATIC elbows – fully extended shoulders at ~70° to 90° wrists				

Co-ordination

Gross Motor ■ control at shoulder, co-ordination between protractors and retractors bilaterally;
■ repetitive movement relying on both sides.

Fine Motor ■ controlled grasp/release.

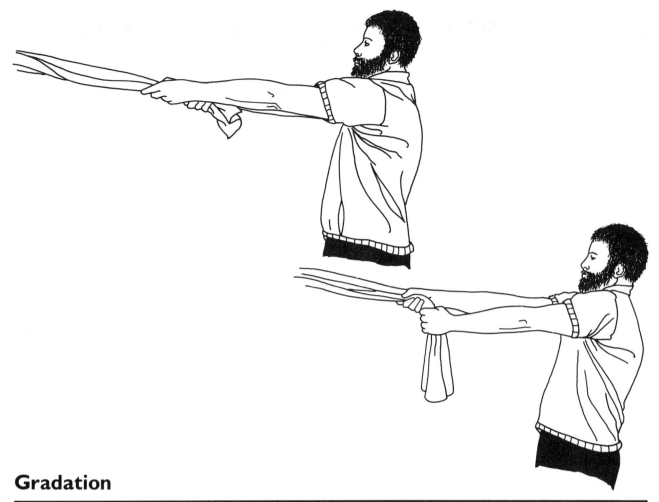

Gradation

	yes/no	How?
RESISTANCE	yes	alter patient position; can be done lying with rope suspended over the shoulders.
RANGE OF MOTION	yes	work within range, starting with small movements and increasing to large ones.
CO-ORDINATION (gross/fine	no	

Also used for:	How?
1 shoulder flex/ext. 2 elbow flex/ext.	suspend rope from ceiling, walk arms up and down rope using shoulder flexion and extension. reach and pull using elbow flexion and extension.

TITLE	**MOVEMENT**
Magic Squares	Shoulder Protraction/Retraction

Category

Purposeful Activity, Light

Description

Patient sits at table with 'magic square' board in front of them. Start with colours, letters or numbers on board in a jumble. Patient sorts the squares into the correct order, moving them with a straight arm, pushing and pulling from the shoulder using shoulder protraction, retraction, horizontal abduction, and horizontal adduction. Palm of hand is open. Alternatively, can have

dowels in the centre of each square and grasp and push the dowels to move the squares (*see Figure 1*).

Equipment

▶ wooden board (21"sq.) with a ¾" rim, fill with 4" × 4" × ⅜" squares (size is optional). Each square has a hole in the centre in which to insert the dowel. Squares can have numbers, letters or colours on them – this can vary on each side of the square (*see Figure 2*). A dowel is also required.

Skills required for activity as exercise
Action

Joints Used	Minimum Jt Range	Main Muscle Groups	Type of Contraction	Minimum Ms Grade
ACTIVE shoulder	full pro/retr.	protractors retractors horiz. abductors horiz. adductors	conc/ecc. ecc/conc. conc/ecc. ecc/conc.	2+ 2+ 2+ 2+
STATIC shoulder flexed to ~70° elbow – fully extended hand – open wrist				

Gross Motor ■ control at shoulder.

Fine Motor ■ if using dowels, sustained grasp is required on the dowel.

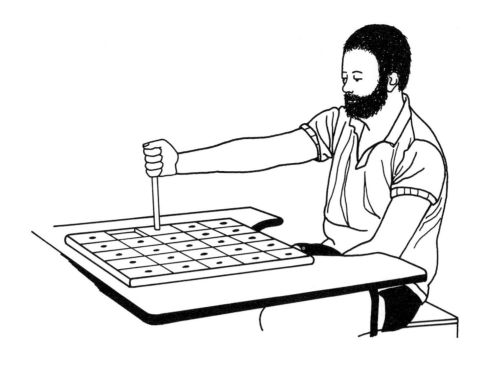

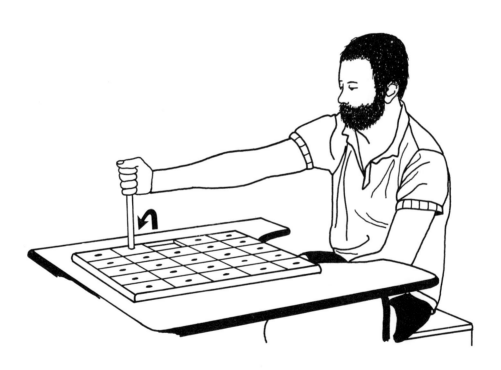

Figure I

Gradation

	yes/no	How?
RESISTANCE	yes	can do on an inclined surface, anti-gravity.
RANGE OF MOTION	yes	alter size and position of board.
CO-ORDINATION (gross/fine)	yes	alter size of squares.

Also used for:	How?
1 elbow flex/ext. 2 shoulder flex/ext. 3 rad/ul. deviation	move squares by flexing and extending elbow. place board on steep angle, such as 45°. use smaller board, move squares with rad/ul. deviation.

Comments

Can be done as a two-handed, active assisted activity by putting a dowel in the centre of each square and grasping the dowel with both hands clasped.

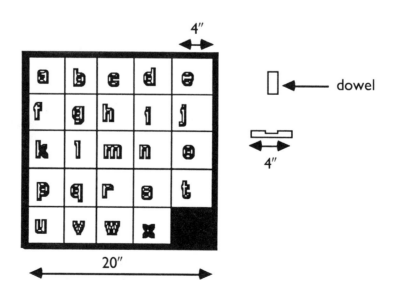

Figure 2

MOVEMENT

Shoulder Horizontal Abduction

Prime Mover

Deltoid (posterior fibres)

Normal Range

see diagram below.

Range of motion:

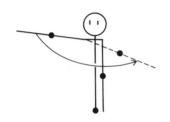

Nerve Supply

Axillary (C$_{5,6}$)

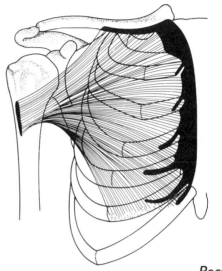

Pectoralis major

MOVEMENT

Shoulder Horizontal Adduction

Prime Movers

Pectoralis Major
(C$_{5,6,7,8}$, T$_1$)

Normal Range

see diagram below.

Range of motion:

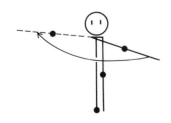

Nerve Supply

Medial and Lateral Pectoral

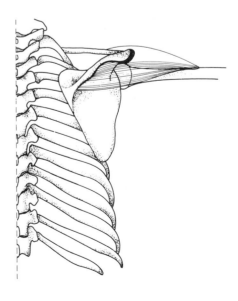

Deltoideus (posterior fibres)

TITLE	MOVEMENT
Dowel Activity	**Shoulder Horizontal Abduction/Adduction**

Category

Therapeutic Exercise, Light

Equipment

▶ 1 × 20″ long, 1″ diameter wooden dowel.

Description

Patient lies supine. With palmar grasp, forearms pronated, and arms straight, hold dowel in air directly in front of shoulders. Swing dowel from side to side, returning to centre over shoulders each time. Repeat as many times as can be tolerated.

Skills required for activity as exercise
Action

Joints Used	Minimum Jt Range	Main Muscle Groups	Type of Contraction	Minimum Ms Grade*
ACTIVE shoulders	~40° mid–range	horiz. abductors horiz. adductors	conc/ecc. (vv) ecc/conc. (vv)	3+ 3+
STATIC elbows – fully extended wrists hands – grasp				

Co-ordination

Gross Motor ■ minimal control at shoulders and elbows;

■ active assisted, bilateral activity – both arms acting in opposite directions simultaneously. Co-ordination required between shoulder horizontal abductors and adductors bilaterally.

Fine Motor ■ sustained grasp.

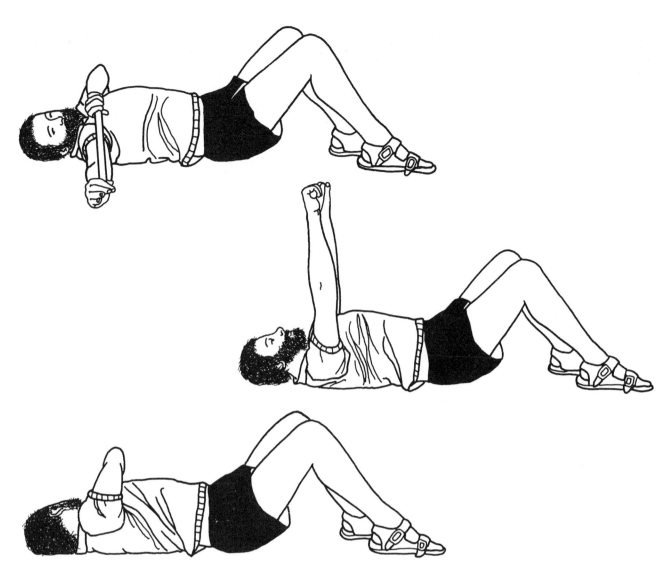

Gradation

	yes/no	How?
RESISTANCE	yes	alter weight of dowel used; place weighted wrist cuffs on patient's wrist.
RANGE OF MOTION	yes	can work within available range.
CO-ORDINATION (gross/fine)	no	

Comments

* This is an active assisted activity. The stronger side can assist the weaker side. It is important that the weaker side has at least grade 3 – in order to participate actively, not just being passively taken through the movement. However, if it is being used as a range of motion exercise, active power on one side may not be necessary, as long as the other side has at least grade 3+ power.

Active participation can be monitored by watching the angle of the dowel (that is, if it sags at one side when held horizontally over shoulders).

TITLE	MOVEMENT
Skateboard	**Shoulder Horizontal Abduction/Adduction**

Category

Therapeutic Exercise, Active Assisted, Light

Description

Patient sits at adjustable height table, table set at about chest height. Place forearm in pronation on 'skateboard', attach straps over wrist and just distal to elbow. Move skateboard across table using horizontal abduction and adduction alternately, moving between two predetermined spots (use large, brightly-coloured dycem spots). Keep elbow extended.

Equipment

▶ 'skateboard' (plastic or wooden platform on four castors with two velcro attaching straps; 2 × 4″ diameter *Dycem* circles.

Skills required for activity as exercise
Action

Joints Used	Minimum Jt Range	Main Muscle Groups	Type of Contraction	Minimum Ms Grade
ACTIVE shoulder	~45° mid-range horiz abd/add.	horiz. abductors horiz. adductors	conc/ecc. ecc/conc.	2– 2–
STATIC elbow – fully extended shoulder at ~70° flexion wrist – relaxed hand – relaxed				

Co-ordination

Gross Motor ■ minimal control at shoulder;
■ ability to move between two targets.

Fine Motor ■ none.

Gradation

	yes/no	How?
RESISTANCE	yes	increase resistance by using an inclined surface; add weights to board.
RANGE OF MOTION	yes	alter distance between targets.
CO-ORDINATION (gross/fine)	yes	can provide lines to follow, or alter size of targets to move to.

Also used for:	How?
1 elbow flex/ext.	move skateboard by using elbow flexion and extension alternately.
2 sh. protraction/ retraction	move skateboard forward and back by thrusting forward and pulling back from shoulder.
3 rad/ul. deviation	use smaller skateboard for hand only; move by using radial and ulnar deviation alternately.

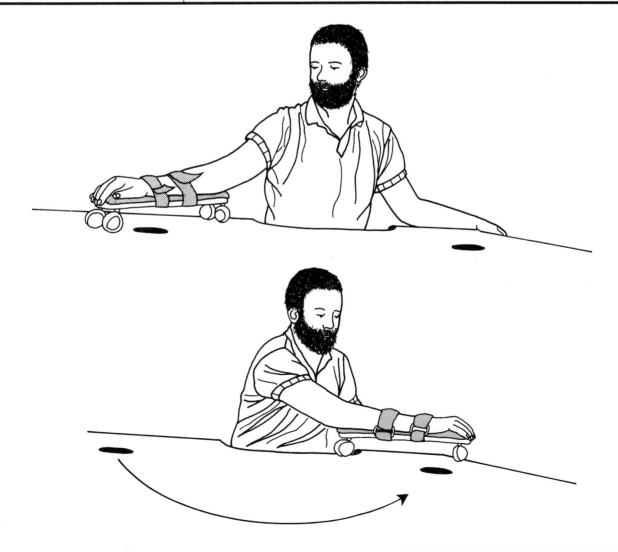

TITLE

Spot Board

MOVEMENT

Shoulder Horizontal Abduction/Adduction

Category

Therapeutic Exercise, Light

Description

Patient sits at table with spot board in front of them. Set up coloured cones on one side of the board. Grasp cones with gross grasp, keep elbow straight, lift, and move them to matching coloured spot on the other side of board (see Figure 1).

Equipment

▶ wooden board of approx. dimensions 40″ × 14″ (see Figure 2);

▶ cones: 5 × red, 5 × yellow, 5 × green (or colours of your choice!).

Skills required for activity as exercise
Action

Joints Used	Minimum Jt Range	Main Muscle Groups	Type of Contraction	Minimum Ms Grade
ACTIVE shoulder	~45° mid-range horiz. abd/add. ~70° flex	horiz. abductors horiz. adductors flexors	conc/ecc. ecc/conc. concentric	2+ 2+ 3+
hand	gross grasp release	flexors extensors	concentric concentric	3+ 3
STATIC elbow – fully extended				

Co-ordination

Gross Motor ■ control at shoulder;
　　　　　　　 ■ accurate targeting and placement.

Fine Motor ■ sustained grasp followed by controlled release.

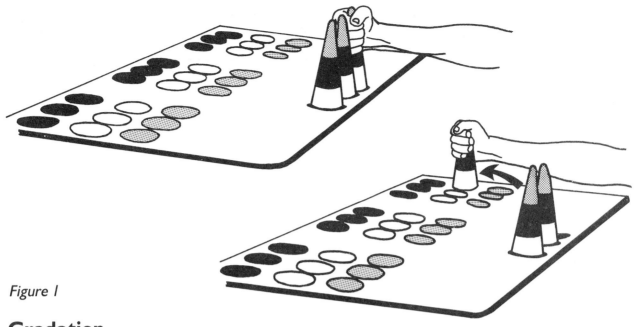

Figure 1

Gradation

	yes/no	How?
RESISTANCE	yes	alter weight of cones or objects moved; place weighted wrist cuffs on patient's wrists.
RANGE OF MOTION	yes	alter targets: can start by moving the cones to adjacent rows; progress to move them across the board to the other side.
CO-ORDINATION (gross/fine)	yes	alter size of target spots.

Also used for:	How?
1 elbow flex/ext.	move cones by bending and straightening elbow.
2 wrist flex/ext.	use smaller board and smaller objects; move objects by flexing and extending wrist.
3 rad/ul. deviation	use smaller board and smaller objects; grasp objects from top, move them by using rad/ul. deviation.

Comments

If one side has less than grade 3+ shoulder flexion, can be done as bilateral active assisted activity, grasping cones with both hands and moving them together.

Board can be adapted for any of the solitaire games.

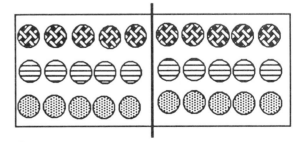

Figure 2

MOVEMENT

Shoulder Extension

Prime Movers

Latissimus Dorsi
Teres Major
Deltoid (posterior fibres)

Normal Range

0° to 50° (beyond mid-line)

Nerve Supply

Thoracodorsal ($C_{6,7,8}$)
Lowest Subscapular ($C_{5,6}$)
Axillary ($C_{5,6}$)

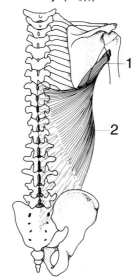

1 Latissimus dorsi

2 Teres major

MOVEMENT

Shoulder Flexion

Prime Movers

Deltoid (anterior fibres)
Coracobrachialis

Normal Range

0° to 90°

Nerve Supply

Axillary ($C_{5,6}$)
Musculocutaneous ($C_{6,7}$)

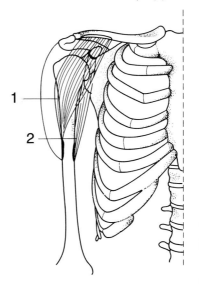

1 Deltoideus
   (anterior fibres)

2 Coracobrachialis

TITLE
Stacking Bricks

MOVEMENT
Shoulder Flexion/ Extension

Category

Therapeutic Exercise, Moderate

Description

Patient stands facing shelves with house bricks placed in front at waist level. Grasp bricks with gross grasp, lift, and place on the shelves in front. Stack as many bricks as possible. Can unstack and restack as much as can be tolerated.

Equipment

▶ adjustable height shelves or table, either freestanding or mounted on wall;

▶ 10 house bricks (or blocks of wood or polystyrene) each of the following weights (or approximations): 75 gr (2.5oz), 300 gr (10oz), 500 gr (1 lb 2.5oz), 600 gr (1 lb 6oz), 2kg 25 gr (4 lb 7.5oz) for gradation.

Skills required for activity as exercise
Action

Joints Used	Minimum Jt Range	Main Muscle Groups	Type of Contraction	Minimum Ms Grade
ACTIVE *Lifting* shoulder hand * elbow	~70° flex gross grasp full ext.	flexors grasp extensors	concentric concentric concentric	4 4 4
Placing and Return shoulder	as above	extensors flexors	concentric eccentric	3
elbow hand	~45° flex. opening	flexors extensors	concentric concentric	3+ 3
STATIC wrist				

Co-ordination

Gross Motor ■ control at shoulder;
■ accurate controlled targeting and placement;
■ ability to stack, good eye/hand co-ordination.

Fine Motor ■ controlled sustained grasp and release.

Gradation

	yes/no	How?
RESISTANCE	yes	alter weight of bricks; place weighted wrist cuffs on patient's wrists.
RANGE OF MOTION	yes	alter target height of shelves.
CO-ORDINATION (gross/fine)	no	

Also used for:	How?
shoulder abd/add.	patient stands sideways to shelves; lifting is achieved using shoulder abduction; return to start by adducting shoulder.

Comments

Can be incorporated into a game of noughts and crosses by painting an X or O on the front of each brick (*see Figure 1*).

Can be incorporated into pre-vocational training where appropriate.

* Watch for over-compensatory movement at elbow (flex/ext.) which would mean not using shoulder flex/ext. to full potential. Avoid this by positioning patient at appropriate distance from target so as to incorporate maximum shoulder flex/ext. available.

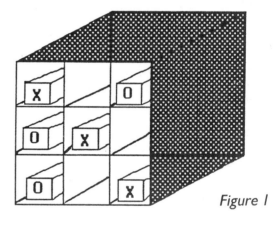

Figure 1

TITLE ■■■■■
Sanding

MOVEMENT ■■■■■
Shoulder Flexion/ Extension

Category

Purposeful Activity, Therapeutic Exercise, Active Assisted, Moderate

Description

Patient stands (sit if necessary) in front of angled, elevated wooden board. Grasp handles at either end of sander, both forearms pronated. Sand wooden board by moving sander up and down with shoulder flexion and extension alternately. Elbows may flex and extend slightly or they can be stabilised with the patient taking a small step back each time the sander is brought down and forward to go up. Can also be done unilaterally.

Equipment

▶ large wooden board;

▶ sanding block, preferably with adaptable handles.

Skills required for activity as exercise
Action

Joints Used	Minimum Jt Range	Main Muscle Groups	Type of Contraction	Minimum Ms Grade
ACTIVE shoulders	~70° mid-range	flexors extensors	*Up.:/Down:* Conc/ecc. ecc/conc.	4 3+
elbows	~20° mid-range	extensors flexors	conc/ecc. ecc/conc.	4 4
STATIC hand elbow wrist				

Co-ordination

Gross Motor ■ control at shoulders and elbows;

■ bilateral activity, both arms working together simultaneously;

■ co-ordination between flexors and extensors for smooth movement.

Fine Motor ■ sustained grasp.

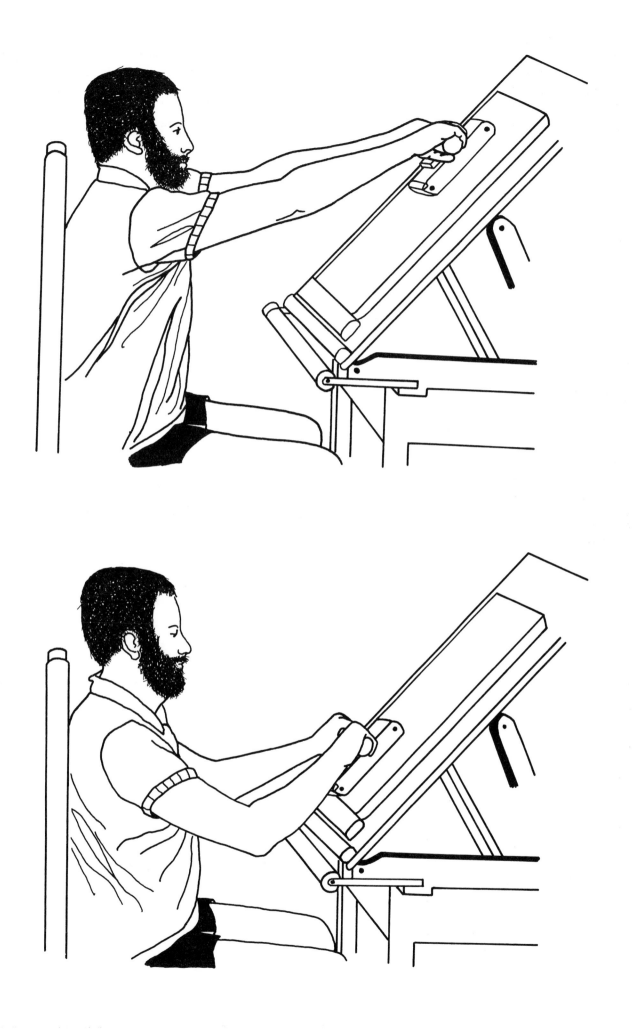

Gradation

	yes/no	How?
RESISTANCE	yes	alter grade of sand paper; apply weighted wrist cuffs to patient; add weights to sander.
RANGE OF MOTION	yes	can start with small movements within shoulder range and increase to larger, longer movements alter angle of board.
CO-ORDINATION (gross/fine)	no	

Also used for:	How?
1 elbow flex/ext.	position patient closer to board; sand by flexing and extending elbows.
2 wrist flex/ext.	add upright dowel handle to top of sander, grasp handles with forearms in neutral, sand by moving sander side to side using wrist flex/ext. alternately.
3 sh. horiz. abd/add.	wooden board flat on table, arms straight, sand by moving sander side to side with horiz. abd/ add.
4 sh. abd/add.	patient stands sideways to board, hold sander in one hand; sand by moving arm up and down (sh. abd/add.) at the side.
5 wrist rad/ul. dev.	hold sander in one hand with palmar grasp, forearm pronated, sand by moving block back and forth using rad. and ul. deviation alternately.

Comments

This can be incorporated into a project where appropriate. This is an active assisted exercise. Therefore, if one side has less than grade 4– shoulder flexors, the other side must have at least grade 4. Watch carefully that patient is not over-compensating with the stronger side and only following passively with the weaker side.

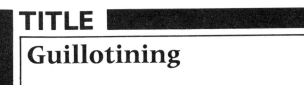

TITLE	MOVEMENT
Guillotining	**Shoulder Flexion/ Extension**

Category

Purposeful Activity, Moderate

Description

Patient stands facing the lever-type paper cutter, at approximately an arm's length away, and paper in place. Reach up, with palmar grasp, grasp the lever, forearm pronated. Pull lever down, keeping arm straight, and when lowering it take a small step back (if unable to step back, can flex at elbow as lowering), slice down through the paper. Paper is stabilised by other hand. Repeat as many times as can be tolerated. Can be done with either arm or both arms simultaneously.

Equipment

▶ 'guillotine' paper cutter that is well stabilised on an adjustable height table;

▶ paper.

Skills required for activity as exercise
Action

Joints Used	Minimum Jt Range	Main Muscle Groups	Type of Contraction	Minimum Ms. Grade
ACTIVE * *Reach Up* shoulder	~45° mid-range	flexors	concentric	3
Pull Down shoulder	same	extensors flexors	concentric eccentric	4-4+
STATIC grasp – palmar elbow – fully extended wrist				

*Only reaching & pulling side analysed; other hand is placing and stabilizing the paper.

Co-ordination

Gross Motor ■ control at shoulder required.

Fine Motor ■ sustained grasp;
■ co-ordination of two hands performing different tasks simultaneously (that is, one hand stabilising paper while other is reaching and pulling lever).

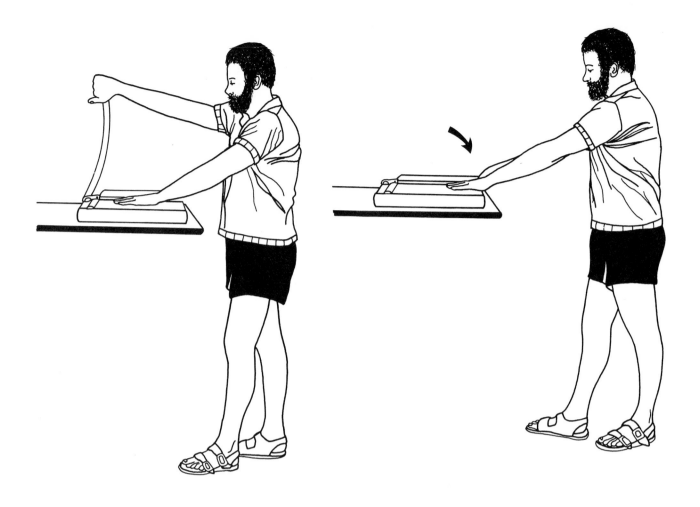

Gradation

	yes/no	How?
RESISTANCE	yes	alter number of pages that are cut at one time; place weighted wrist cuffs on patient's wrists.
RANGE OF MOTION	yes	alter length of lever (that is, to increase range required increase length of lever); alter height of table.
CO-ORDINATION (gross/fine)	no	

Also used for:	How?
1 shoulder add/abd.	patient stands sideways to paper cutter, reaches up using shoulder abduction and pulls down using shoulder adduction.
2 elbow ext/flex.	patient stands closer to paper cutter, reaches up using shoulder flex and elbow ext, pulls down using elbow flexion.

Comments

This activity can be used purely as an exercise or can be incorporated into a functional or pre-vocational task if appropriate.

Can adapt grasp with 'C–Clip' (see below) or built up handle. C-CLIP HANDLE: An adaptation that can be fabricated out of a thermoplastic material such as sansplint and is attached to the handle. It goes through the webspace and over the dorsum of the hand (see diagram below).

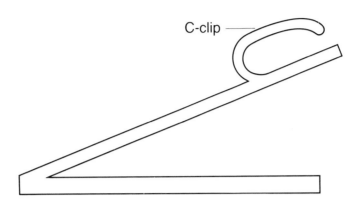

C-clip

■ TITLE ■■■■
Chopping

MOVEMENT ■■■■
Shoulder Extension/ Flexion

Category

Therapeutic Exercise, Active Assisted, Light

Equipment

▶ wooden dowel.

Description

Patient sits or stands. Clasp hands together or grasp dowel in both hands, forearms in mid-position. Raise both arms over the head, then with chopping action lower them down towards knees. Keep arms straight throughout.

Skills required for activity as exercise
Action

Joints Used	Minimum Jt Range	Main Muscle Groups	Type of Contraction	Minimum Ms Grade
ACTIVE *Lifting* shoulder	30° mid-range	flexors	concentric	3*
Chopping shoulder	~15°	extensors flexors	concentric eccentric	0 (can let gravity assist)
Both hands	gross grasp	grasp	concentric	3+
STATIC wrist elbow				

Co-ordination

Gross Motor ■ control at shoulder;
■ co-ordination between shoulder flexors and extensors for smooth chopping and lifting action.

Fine Motor ■ sustained grasp.

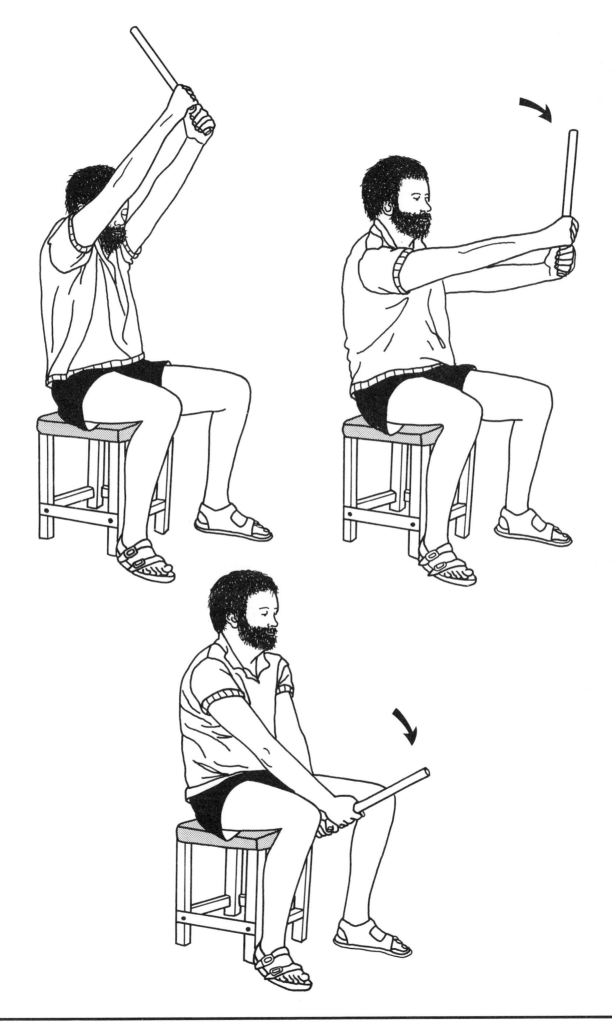

Gradation

	yes/no	How?
RESISTANCE	yes	alter weight of dowel: either add weights to each end or vary the weights of the dowels used; place weighted wrist cuffs on patient.
RANGE OF MOTION	yes	can work within available range starting at approx. 30°; watch that patient is not using trunk to compensate for lack of range in shoulder.
CO-ORDINATION (gross/fine)	no	

Also used for:	How?
horiz. abd/add.	grasp dowel with both hands either in pronation or supination, swing arms from side to side with shoulders flexed to 90°.

Comments

*This is an active assisted activity, the stronger arm may assist the weaker one. Watch carefully that the weaker is not just following passively, it must actively assist. Therefore, if one side has less than grade 3 shoulder flexion, the other must have at least grade 3+ − 4. For chopping action, arms can be brought down by gravity. However, the aim is to use a controlled action with co-ordination between shoulder flexors and extensors acting eccentrically and concentrically. Can be incorporated into functional activity of chopping wood where appropriate. Must be done under close supervision.

MOVEMENT

Shoulder Abduction

Prime Movers

Deltoid (middle fibres)

Supraspinatus

Normal Range

0° to 90°

Nerve Supply

Axillary ($C_{5,6}$)

Suprascapular (C_5)

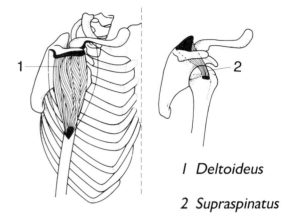

1 *Deltoideus*

2 *Supraspinatus*

MOVEMENT

Shoulder Adduction

Prime Movers

Pectoralis Major

Latissimus Dorsi

Long Head Triceps

Teres Major

Normal Range

90° to 0°

Nerve Supply

Medial and Lateral Pectoral ($C_{5,6,7,8}$,T_1)

Thoracodorsal ($C_{6,7,8}$)

Radial ($C_{7,8}$)

Lowest Subscapular ($C_{5,6}$)

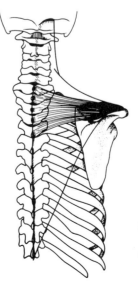

Posterior View

Trapezius (middle fibres)

<table>
<tr><td>

TITLE

Br"ntease (Solitaire)

</td><td>

MOVEMENT

Shoulder Abduction/ Adduction

</td></tr>
</table>

Category

Purposeful Activity, Light

Description

Patient stands or sits positioned sideways to large 'braintease' board. Start with board set up as in Figure 1 with one vacant spot. Move by jumping ball over another ball into a vacant spot; remove the ball that was jumped. The object is to leave one ball on the board. Reaching for and moving the balls is achieved by using shoulder abduction and adduction alternately, and slight elbow flexion

and extension alternately. Can be done with both sides by getting patient to turn around.

Equipment

▶ large triangular 'braintease' board with 15 tennis balls attached with velcro, (*see Figure 1 for dimensions and set-up*).

Skills required for activity as exercise
Action

Joints Used	Minimum Jt Range	Main Muscle Groups	Type of Contraction	Minimum Ms Grade
ACTIVE *Reach & Jump* shoulder elbow	~70° abd/add. full ext. ~45° flex.	abductors extensors flexors	concentric conc/ecc. ecc/conc.	3+ 3+ 3+
hand	full grasp/rel.	grasp/release	conc/ecc. (vv)	3+
Remove & Put Down shoulder	as above	adductors abductors	concentric eccentric	0*
hand (as above)				
STATIC wrist				

Co-ordination

Gross Motor ■ control at shoulder;
■ accurate targeting and placement.

Fine Motor ■ controlled sustained grasp with timed release.

Gradation

	yes/no	How?
RESISTANCE	yes	alter type and weight of pieces and attachment method (eg. large pegs attached by insertion into holes, weighted balls); place weighted wrist cuffs on patient's wrists.
RANGE OF MOTION	yes	alter height and position of board.
CO-ORDINATION (gross/fine)	yes	alter 'pieces' and attachment method (eg. pegs that insert into small holes require more accurate targeting & placement than velcro attaching balls).

Also used for:	How?
I shoulder flex/ext.	patient stands or sits facing board; reach for balls using shoulder flexion, bring them down with shoulder extension.

Comment

*Patients lacking active hand function can use disks with 'C-clips' attached; patient slips hand through.

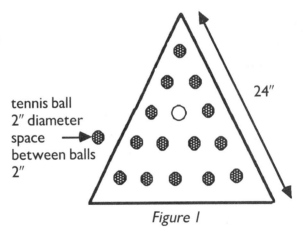

tennis ball 2" diameter

space ➝ between balls 2"

24"

Figure I

TITLE ▮▮▮▮▮▮▮▮

Finger Ladder

MOVEMENT ▮▮▮▮▮▮

Shoulder Abduction

Category

Therapeutic Exercise, Light

Description

Patient sits or stands sideways to finger ladder that is mounted on the wall (*see Figure 1*) or free-standing on a table (*see Figure 2*). Start at lowest rung (within available range) and walk fingers up the ladder to the highest rung possible. Either walk fingers back down again or bring down to side in a slow, controlled fashion. Keep elbow straight throughout. Repeat with each arm as many times as possible.

Equipment

▶ small ladder mounted on adjustable height wall bracket, or free-standing and clamped to a table. Each rung about 2–3″ apart and numbered so that patient can record progress.

Skills required for activity as exercise
Action

Joints Used	Minimum Jt Range	Main Muscle Groups	Type of Contraction	Minimum Ms Grade
ACTIVE *Climbing* shoulder fingers	~45°–90° partial ROM	abductors flexors/extensors	concentric conc/ecc. (vv)	3− 3
Returning shoulder	as above	adductors abductors	concentric eccentric	0–3
fingers	(as above or inactive)			
STATIC elbow – fully extended wrist				

Co-ordination

Gross Motor ■ control at shoulder;
■ can externally stabilise elbow if necessary.

Fine Motor ■ the fine motor control of fingers, co-ordination between flexors and extensors as they climb ladder.

Gradation

	yes/no	How?
RESISTANCE	yes	place weighted wrist cuffs on patient's wrists.
RANGE OF MOTION	yes	can work within available range, note number of rung achieved each time; watch that patient does not compensate for lack of shoulder range with lateral trunk movement.
CO-ORDINATION (gross/fine)	no	

Also used for	How?
1 shoulder flexion 2 finger flex/ext.	patient stands facing finger ladder; walks fingers up ladder, keeping elbow straight, using shoulder flexion. patient sits close to finger ladder, forearm pronated; walk fingers up and down ladder as many times as can be tolerated.

Comments

This is an active assisted activity, therefore if patient has less than grade 3 abductors, fingers will assist. However, they must have a minimum of grade 3 – for activity to be effective, otherwise they may be fully supporting arm with fingers.

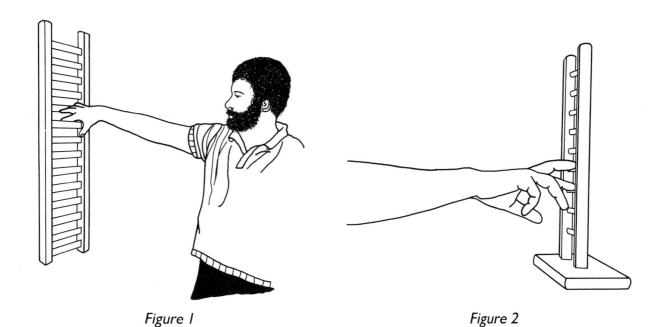

Figure 1   Figure 2

TITLE
Dowel Activity

MOVEMENT
Shoulder Abduction/ Adduction

Category

Therapeutic Exercise, Light

Equipment

▶ 1 × 20″ long, 1″ diameter wooden dowel.

Description

Patient stands. With palmar grasp, forearms pronated, and arms straight, hold dowel down in front of thighs. Swing dowel from side to side, returning to centre at thigh level each time. Swing arms as high as possible each time and repeat as many times as can be tolerated.

Skills required for activity as exercise
Action

Joints Used	Minmum Jt Range	Main Muscle Groups	Type of Contraction	Minimum Ms Grade*
ACTIVE shoulders	~40° mid-range	abductors adductors int. rotators	conc/ecc. (vv) ecc/conc. (vv) concentric	3— 3— 3—
elbows	full ext. to ~ 85° flex	flexors extensors	conc/ecc. (vv) ecc/conc. (vv)	3— 3
STATIC wrists hands – grasp				

Co-ordination

Gross Motor ■ minimal control at shoulders and elbows;

■ active assisted, bilateral activity – both arms acting in opposite directions simultaneously. Co-ordination required between shoulder abductors and adductors bilaterally.

Fine Motor ■ sustained grasp.

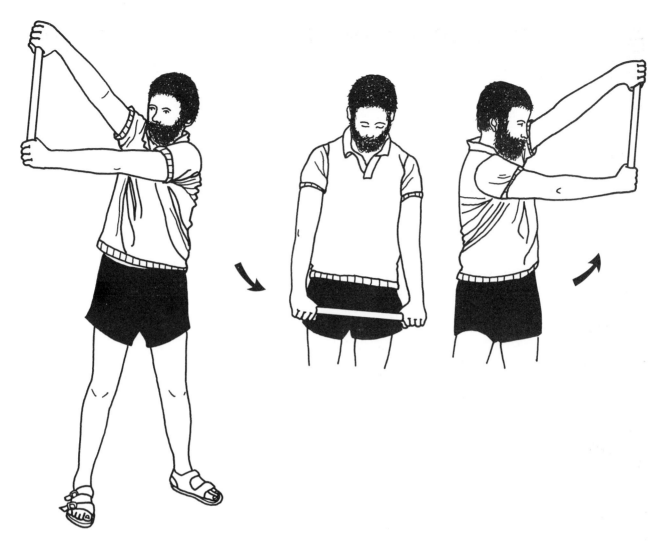

Gradation

	yes/no	How?
RESISTANCE	yes	alter weight of dowel used; place weighted wrist cuffs on patient's wrists.
RANGE OF MOTION	yes	can work within available range.
CO-ORDINATION (gross/fine)	no	

Comments

* This is an active assisted activity. Therefore, if one side is weaker, the stronger side can assist. It is important that the weaker side has at least grade 3— in order to participate actively, not just being passively taken through the movement. However, if it is being used as a range of motion exercise, active power is not necessary on the weaker side.

TITLE

Pyramids

MOVEMENT

Shoulder Abduction/ Adduction

Category

Purposeful Activity, Light

Description

Patient sits at table with 'pyramid' game beside them an arm's length away. To start, the disks are stacked in order, largest at the bottom, and placed on any dowel. The object is to rebuild the pyramid on one of the other dowels, never putting a larger disk on top of a smaller one, and only moving one at a time. To complete this task may take up to a hundred or more separate moves. The patient picks up the disk between thumb and fingers, forearm supinated, and elbow straight. Lift disk off the dowel using shoulder abduction and place it on the chosen dowel using shoulder adduction.

Equipment

▶ wooden base with three vertical dowels spaced ~3½″ apart; the dowels should be height adjustable — either wooden dowels of varying heights that can be inserted into the three holes or telescopic tubing (eg. radio antenna), 3″–42″.

▶ Five disks with a hole in the middle of each (large enough to fit over the dowels); the disks start at 3½″ diameter and decrease in size by ½″ each, the fifth one being 1½″. The size of the disks, dowels and space between dowels can all be altered.

Skills required for activity as exercise
Action

Joints Used	Minimum Jt Range	Main Muscle Groups	Type of Contraction	Minimum Ms Grade
ACTIVE *Lift* shoulder	~40 mid-range	abductors	concentric	3+
Placement shoulder	as above	adductors abductors	concentric eccentric	3
Both hand	partial finger flex/ext.	flexors/extensors	conc/ecc. (vv)	3+
STATIC elbow – extended wrist				

Co-ordination

Gross Motor ■ control at shoulder;
■ accurate targeting and placement, good eye/hand co-ordination.

Fine Motor ■ controlled sustained grasp followed by controlled, accurate release.

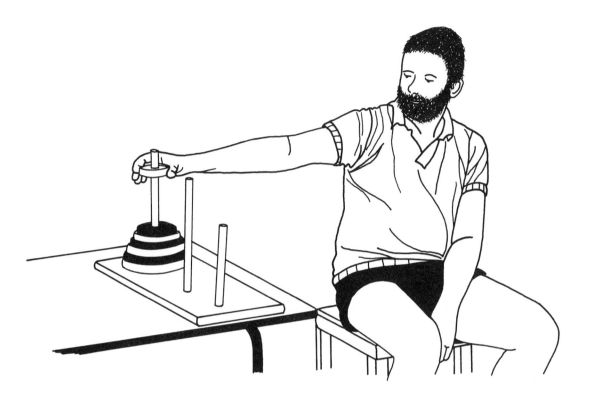

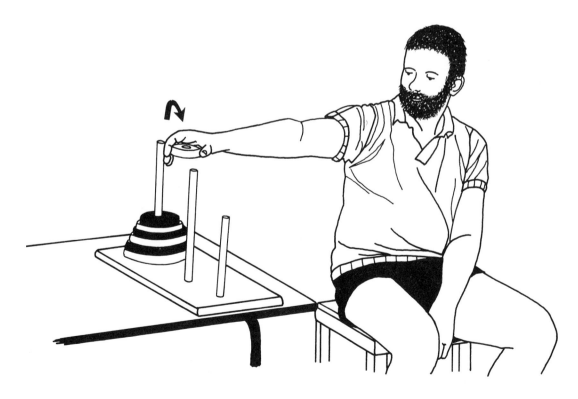

Gradation

	yes/no	How?
RESISTANCE	yes	alter size and weight of disks; place weighted wrist cuffs on patient.
RANGE OF MOTION	yes	alter height of dowels or tubing.
CO-ORDINATION (gross/fine)	yes	alter size of hole in disk and diameter of dowel (smaller hole and dowel requires finer control); alter diameter of disk – larger disk requires grosser grasp.

Also used for:	How?
1 shoulder flex/ext.	patient stands or sits facing game; lift disks using shoulder flex. replace using shoulder ext.
2 elbow flex/ext.	patient faces game with it positioned closed; use elbow flex/ext. alternately to lift and replace disks.
3 pronation/supination	hold arm at side, elbow flexed to ~90°; lift disks with forearm supinated, pronate, and replace in pronation.
4 shoulder rotation	same positioning as for shoulder flex/ext., lift disk from underneath with arm externally rotated and forearm supinated, turn over and replace with arm internally rotated and forearm pronated.
5 tenodesis training	grasp disks using tenodesis grasp, release by flexing wrist.

Comments

For those lacking active hand function, add wire loops to sides of the disks, patient then inserts thumb into loop. Grasp can be altered as appropriate for picking up the disks.

MOVEMENT

Shoulder Internal Rotation

Prime Movers

Subscapularis
Pectoralis Major
Latissimus Dorsi
Teres Major

Normal Range

0° to 90°

Nerve Supply

Upper and Lower Subscapular ($C_{5,6}$)
Medial and Lateral Pectoral ($C_{5,6,7,8}$,T_1)
Thoracodorsal ($C_{6,7,8}$)
Lowest Subscapular ($C_{5,6}$)

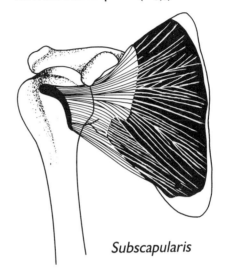

Subscapularis

MOVEMENT

Shoulder External Rotation

Prime Movers

Infraspinatus
Teres Minor

Normal Range

0° to 90°

Nerve Supply

Suprascapular ($C_{5,6}$)
Axillary (C_5)

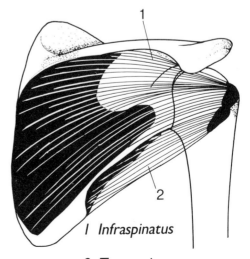

1 Infraspinatus

2 Teres minor

TITLE ■
Dowel – Rotation

MOVEMENT ■
Shoulder Rotation

Category

Therapeutic Exercise, Light (Active Assisted)

Equipment

▶ several 15″ dowels of varying weights (for gradation).

Description

Patient sits or stands. Grasp 15″ dowel with palmar grasp, one hand above the other and close together, dowel in upright position, elbows straight. Hold dowel out in front and make small semi-circles, first clockwise and then anti-clockwise.

Skills required for activity as exercise
Action

Joints Used	Minimum Jt Range	Main Muscle Groups	Type of Contraction	Minimum Ms Grade
ACTIVE shoulder	~$\frac{1}{2}$ rot. bilaterally	rotators (alternately)	conc/ecc. (vv)	3
STATIC shoulder at ~90° flex elbow – fully extended wrist hand – grasp				

Co-ordination

Gross Motor ■ control at shoulders, co-ordination between rotators;
■ co-ordinated action between two arms working in opposite directions.

Fine Motor ■ sustained grasp.

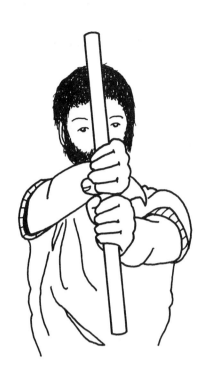
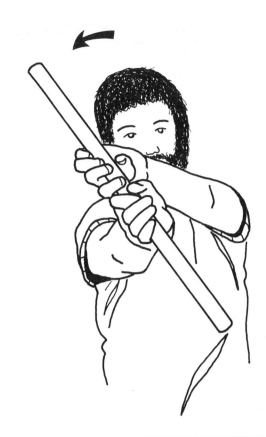

Gradation

	yes/no	How?
RESISTANCE	yes	alter weight of dowel used; place weighted wrist cuffs on patient's wrists.
RANGE OF MOTION	yes	can work within available range, starting with partial arcs and going to almost complete circles.
CO-ORDINATION (gross/fine)	no	

Also used for:	How?
pronation/supination	hold elbows at side and flex them to 90°, grasp dowel with palmar grasp in centre of dowel, hands close together. Make semi-circles with dowel using pronation/supination alternately.

Comments

For those lacking active grasp dowel can be adapted with 'C-clips' or strap handles in appropriate place.

If a computer is available, flat switches can be set up at either side of forearms. Use the dowel as described to activate the switches while playing a computer game. This may enhance motivation.

TITLE	MOVEMENT
Stick Printing	**Shoulder Rotation**

Category

Purposeful Activity, Light

Description

Patient sits at table with paper in front. Have ink pads mounted vertically at each side, an arm's length away (*see Figure 1*). Grasp the printing block handle with a gross palmar grasp, hold arm in an extended position. Stamp printing block on the mounted ink pad; forearm is pronated and shoulder flexed. Bring arm across to paper, internally rotate shoulder and stamp block on paper. Then fully externally rotate shoulder to stamp ink pad on opposite side and fully internally rotate to stamp paper again. Repeat whole routine as many times as can be tolerated.

Equipment

► rubber ink stamps with 4″ long handles, pads mounted on side walls;

► paper on adjustable height table.

Skills required for activity as exercise
Action

Joints Used	Minimum Jt Range	Main Muscle Groups	Type of Contraction	Minimum Ms Grade
ACTIVE shoulder	full rotation ~90° mid-range	rotators horiz. abductors and adductors	conc/ecc. (vv) conc/ecc. (vv) conc/ecc. (vv)	3+ 3 3+
	~80° flex.	flexors extensors	ecc/conc. (vv)	
STATIC hand (gross grasp) elbow (fully extended)				

Co-ordination

Gross Motor ■ control at shoulder;
■ co-ordinated action between internal and external rotators.

Fine Motor ■ sustained grasp.

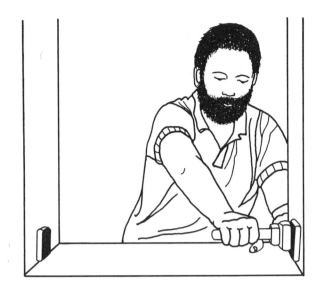
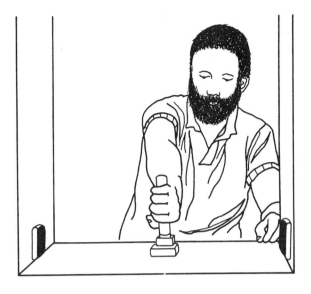
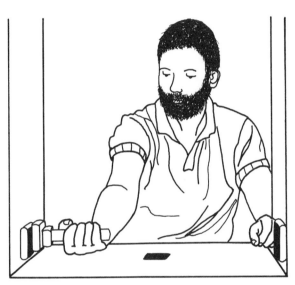

Figure 1

Gradation

	yes/no	How?
RESISTANCE	yes	use stamps of varying weights; place weighted wrist cuffs on patient's wrists.
RANGE OF MOTION	yes	alter positioning of paper and pad.
CO-ORDINATION (gross/fine)	yes	alter size of ink pad and paper; for finer control can set smaller target area.

Also used for:	How?
1 pron/sup.	hold arm at side, alter placement of pad and paper, elbow flexed to 90°; stamping action achieved with pronation/supination alternately.
2 wrist flex/ext.	place rubber stamp on wall in front of paper, adapt handle with bar (*see Figure 2*). Rest forearm on 'ski jump' support. Use wrist flex/ext. alternately to stamp pad and paper.
3 shoulder flex/ext.	mount paper or ink pad at shoulder height in front of patient, use shoulder flex/ext. alternately to stamp pad and paper.
4 shoulder abd/add.	using same stamp as in (2), place paper on wall at side and at shoulder height of patient; use shoulder abd/add. alternately for stamping.

Comments

For those lacking active hand function, adapt handle with cross bar type handle (see diagram); Can also adapt handle with ball grip, built-up grip and so on. Printing stamps can be readily purchased.

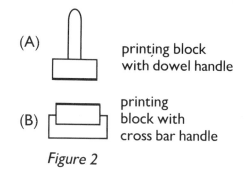

(A) printing block with dowel handle

(B) printing block with cross bar handle

Figure 2

TITLE

Suspended Ball Activity

MOVEMENT

Shoulder Rotation

Category

Therapeutic Exercise, Light

Description

Patient sits in front of suspended ball, arm held at side, and elbow flexed to 90°. Hit ball, first with palm and then with dorsum of hand, rotating at the shoulder each time. Can also be done using a paddle to hit the ball.

Equipment

▶ adjustable height suspension from ceiling with hook attachment at the bottom on which to hang the appropriate size and weight of ball; various sizes and weights of balls, with an attachment hook.

Skills required for activity as exercise
Action

Joints Used	Minimum Jt Range	Main Muscle Groups	Type of Contraction	Minimum Ms Grade
ACTIVE shoulder	~ 70° rotation	rotators	conc/ecc. (vv)	3+
STATIC elbow – flexed to 90° hand – opened shoulder – adducted				

Co-ordination

Gross Motor ■ control at shoulder and trunk;
■ accurate timing to hit the ball.

Fine Motor ■ sustained open hand.

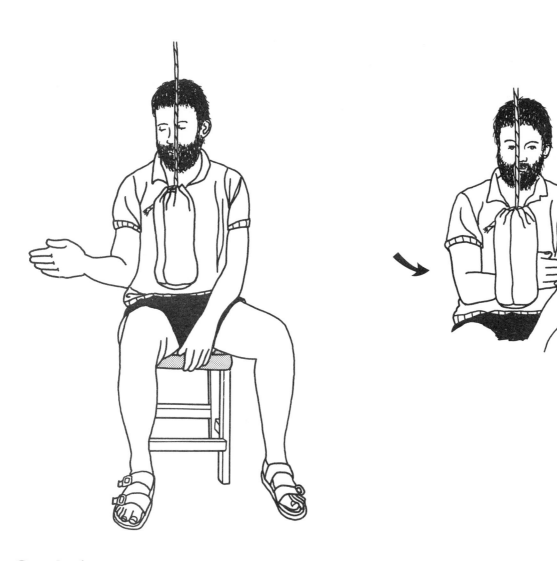

Gradation

	yes/no	How?
RESISTANCE	yes	alter the weight of ball (eg. balloon, beach ball, plastic ball, rubber ball, solid ball).
RANGE OF MOTION	yes	work within available range; start with small short hits and progress to larger hits.
CO-ORDINATION (gross/fine)	yes	alter size of ball (larger ball requires less accurate timing and control).

Also used for:	How?
1 shoulder horiz. abd/add.	hold arm straight out at shoulder height, hit ball by bringing arm straight across body and out again.
2 elbow flex/ext.	hit ball by straightening and bending elbow.
3 shoulder protr/retra.	punch ball, thrusting forward from shoulder, with elbows straight.

MOVEMENT

Elbow Flexion

Prime Movers

Biceps Brachii

Brachialis

Brachioradialis

Normal Range

0° to 145° – 165°

Nerve Supply

Musculotaneous (C$_{5,6}$)

Musculotaneous (C$_{5,6}$)

Radial (C$_{5,6}$)

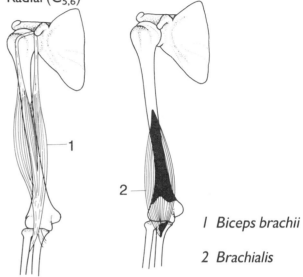

1 *Biceps brachii*

2 *Brachialis*

MOVEMENT

Elbow Extension

Prime Movers

Triceps Brachii

Normal Range

145° – 165° to 0°

Nerve Supply

Radial (C$_{7,8}$)

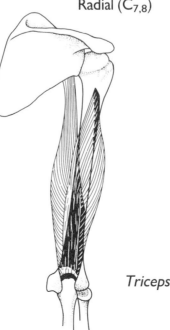

Triceps brachii

TITLE ∎
Knights (form of solitaire)

MOVEMENT ∎
Elbow Flexion/ Extension

Category

Purposeful Activity, Light

Description

Set out board as in Figure 1, leaving centre empty. Using the 'knight's move' as in chess, transpose the white and black knights. A 'knight's move' is either one forward and two sideways or two forward and one sideways in any direction to land in an empty space. Patient sits (or can stand) in front of board mounted on the wall, an arm's length away. Grasp knights in hand and remove using elbow flexion; place by extending the elbow.

Equipment

▶ large square board with five rows and five columns of either holes or circular velcro pieces evenly spaced apart (see Figure 1);

▶ 12 white and 12 black 'knights' (as in chess) with either pegs or velcro on the bottom for attachment (see Figure 1);

▶ adjustable mounting equipment for wall or adjustable angle, table-top stand.

Skills required for activity as exercise
Action

Joints Used	Minimum Jt Range	Main Muscle Groups	Type of Contraction	Minimum Ms Grade
ACTIVE *Remove*				
elbow	~45° flex.	flexors	concentric	3+
shoulder	~110° flex.	flexors	concentric	3+
hand	gross grasp	grasp	concentric	3+
Reach and Replace				
elbow	~20° ext.	extensors flexors	concentric eccentric	3−
shoulder	as above	extensors flexors	concentric eccentric	3−
hand	partial opening	release	concentric	3

Co-ordination

Gross Motor ∎ control at shoulder and elbow;
∎ accurate targeting and placement;
∎ controlled, repetitive movement.

Fine Motor ∎ controlled grasp (sustained) then release.

Gradation

	yes/no	How?
RESISTANCE	yes	alter positioning of board (eg. place board on table); alter attachment method (with varying stiffness of velcro, peg attachment) – *see Figure 1 below*; alter size and weight of 'knights' or use wrist cuffs.
RANGE OF MOTION	yes	alter position of board from patient; alter height of 'knights'.
CO-ORDINATION (gross/fine)	yes	alter size and attachment method of 'knights' (eg. large 'knights' attached by large velcro require less motor control than small ones attached by pegs).

Also used for:	How?
1 shoulder flex/ext.	same technique as above but with more emphasis on shoulder movement.
2 shoulder abd/add.	patient is positioned sideways to board; remove and replace 'knights' using shoulder abduction and adduction.
3 shoulder prot/retr.	using straight arm, reach for 'knights' using protraction; pull out using retraction.
4 tenodesis training	grasp 'knights' using tenodesis action.

Comments

Patient must be made aware of therapeutic goal of exercise and encouraged not to take a long time over each move. Score is not important, whereas repetitive movement is.

For those lacking active grasp and tenodesis action, 'knights' can be adapted with loops or cuffs.

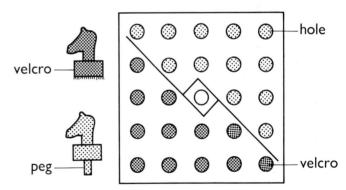

Figure 1

TITLE
Shove Board

MOVEMENT
Elbow Flexion/ Extension

Category

Purposeful Activity, Light

Description

Patient stands or sits in front of shove board.

Flexion: Patient is sideways to board. Push disk towards target using a quick movement of elbow flexion. The aim is to get disk into target with highest numerical value.

Extension: Patient faces board, palm over disk. Push disk towards target by quick straightening of the elbow (elbow extension) – *see Figure 1*.

Equipment

▶ shove board (*see Figure 2 for dimensions*) ; can have targets that are numerically valued (aim to score highest points), colours (aim to match same coloured disk to target), numbers (match numbers) and so on.

Skills required for activity as exercise
Action

Joints Used	Minimum Jt Range	Main Muscle Groups	Type of Contraction	Minimum Ms Grade
ACTIVE *Flexion* elbow	~60°	flexors extensors	concentric eccentric	3−
STATIC shoulder at ~70–90°				
ACTIVE *Extension* elbow	~60°	extensors flexors	concentric eccentric	3−
STATIC shoulder at ~90°				
Both hand	loose palmar grasp	grasp/release	conc/ecc. (vv)	3+

Co-ordination

Gross Motor ■ shoulder and elbow control;
■ accurate targeting, good eye/
hand co-ordination.

Fine Motor ■ loose palmar grasp with co-
ordinated and timely release.

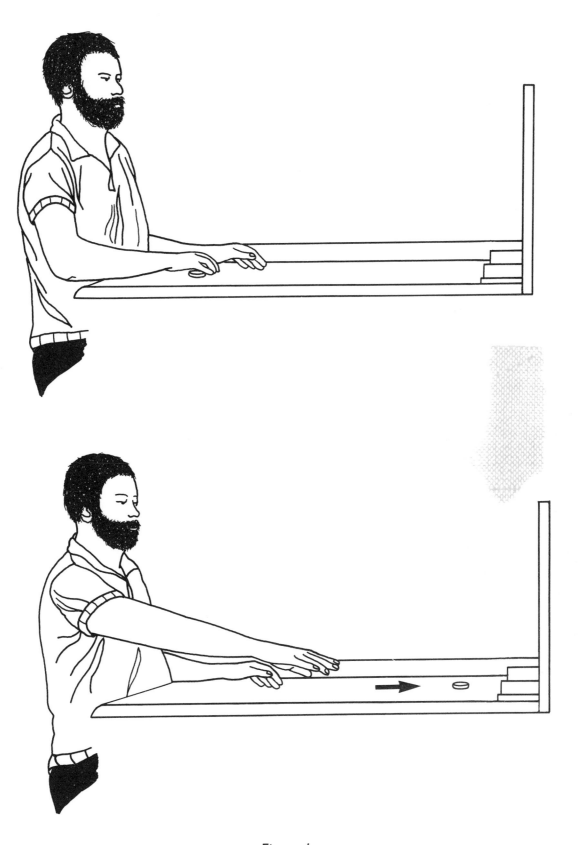

Figure 1

Gradation

	yes/no	How?
RESISTANCE	yes	alter size and weight of disks (eg. use wood, metal, or plastic); alter length of board – greater length requires greater push.
RANGE OF MOTION	yes	can work within available range starting at approx. 60°.
CO-ORDINATION (gross/fine)	yes	alter size of disks and size of targets.

Also used for:	How?
1 rad/ul. deviation	stabilise elbow, grasp disks in palm, forearm pronated; pull back and release disk with a flick at the wrist using radial/ulnar deviation.
2 shoulder horiz. add/abd.	stand or sit sideways to board, hold arm straight, use horizontal adduction to push.

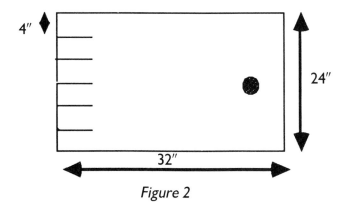

Figure 2

There is a commercially made 'shove board' available.

MOVEMENT

Forearm Pronation

Prime Movers

Pronator Teres

Pronator Quadratus

Normal Range

0° to 90° (from mid-position)

Nerve Supply

Median ($C_{6,7}$)

Median (C_8,T_1)

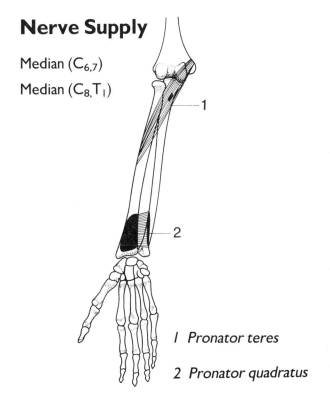

1 Pronator teres

2 Pronator quadratus

MOVEMENT

Forearm Supination

Prime Movers

Biceps Brachii

Supinator

Normal Range

0° to 90° (from mid-position)

Nerve Supply

Musculocutaneous ($C_{5,6}$)

Radial (C_6)

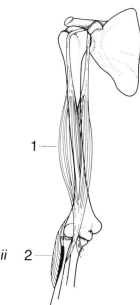

1 Biceps brachii

2 Supinator

TITLE

Pronation/Supination Dowel

MOVEMENT

Pronation/Supination

Category

Therapeutic Exercise, Light

Equipment

▶ 10″ dowels of varying weights (alternatively, use a hammer or mallet);

▶ 'ski jump'.

Description

Patient sits with arm at side and elbow flexed to 90°, arm supported on a 'ski jump'; hold dowel in the centre with forearm in mid-position. In a slow, controlled manner turn it palm down and then palm up. Do as many repetitions as can be tolerated.

Skills required for activity as exercise
Action

Joints Used	Minimum Jt Range	Main Muscle Groups	Type of Contraction	Minimum Ms Grade
ACTIVE rad/ul. joints.	$\sim\frac{1}{4}$	pronators supinators	conc/ecc. (vv) ecc/conc. (vv)	3+ 3+
hand	gross grasp	grasp	concentric	3+
STATIC elbow at ~90°				

Co-ordination

Gross Motor ■ forearm + wrist control;
■ controlled repetitive movement.

Fine Motor ■ sustained grasp.

Gradation

	yes/no	How?
RESISTANCE	yes	alter weight of dowels (can either have dowels of varying weights or add weights to ends); start with just pure movement, no dowel.
RANGE OF MOTION	yes	work within available range starting at $\sim\frac{1}{4}$. NB. a weighted dowel can encourage increase in ROM.
CO-ORDINATION (gross/fine)	yes	if affected arm lacks co-ordinated movement, grasp dowel with both hands to assist with unaffected side.

Also used for:	How?
shoulder rotation	do with straight arm and turn from shoulder using shoulder rotation.

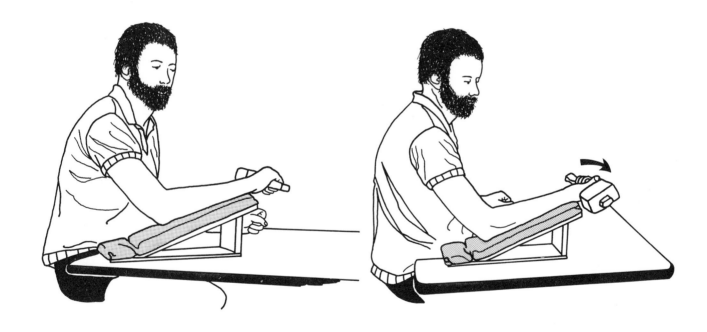

TITLE
Wire Maze

MOVEMENT
Pronation/ Supination

Category

Therapeutic Exercise, Light

Description

Grasp handle attached to the wire maze. Hold arm in at side with elbow flexed to 90°. Move bead from one side of handle to the other by using wrist movement – primarily pronation and supination alternately. Can record time taken if appropriate.

Equipment

▶ wire mazes of varying complexity attached to wooden handles;

▶ one bead that moves freely over wire.

Skills required for activity as exercise
Action

Joints Used	Minimum Jt Range	Main Muscle Groups	Type of Contraction	Minimum Ms Grade
ACTIVE rad/ul. joints.	$\sim\frac{3}{4}$	pronators supinators	conc/ecc. (vv) ecc/conc. (vv)	3+ 3+
wrist	$\sim\frac{3}{4}$	flexors extensors	conc/ecc. (vv) ecc/conc. (vv)	3+ 3+
hand	full gross grasp	grasp	concentric	3+
STATIC elbow at 90° shoulder (watch carefully that movement is not coming from shoulder)				

Co-ordination

Gross Motor ■ control at forearm and wrist;
■ requires intact motor praxia (motor planning).

Fine Motor ■ sustained grasp.

Gradation

	yes/no	How?
RESISTANCE	yes	alter size and weight of wire maze.
RANGE OF MOTION	yes	alter complexity and distance of wire between start and finish points.
CO-ORDINATION (gross/fine)	yes	alter complexity of wire maze.

Also used for:	How?
1 shoulder IR/ER	do not hold arm at side; use shoulder IR/ER to move bead. Can also use board with wire attached. Hold in hands at either end and move by using shoulder IR/ER.
2 wrist flex/ext.	same technique as for pron/sup. but primarily using wrist flex/ext.

Comments

Wire mazes are commercially available.

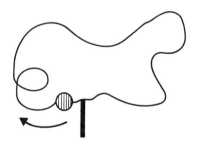

TITLE
Threaded Solitaire I

MOVEMENT
Pronation/ Supination

Category

Purposeful Activity, Moderate

Description

Patient sits or stands in front of large solitaire board that is mounted at chest height. Patient plays solitaire by unscrewing one wheel, jumping, and screwing it into a vacant spot. Then remove the wheel that was jumped by unscrewing it. To remove and replace wheels, grasp the wheel with palmar grasp and twist it by using pronation or supination depending on the direction required. Keep elbow close to side.

Equipment

▶ large solitaire board with screw-on wheels as pieces;

▶ adjustable height and angled mounting bracket.

Skills required for activity as exercise
Action

Joints Used	Minimum Jt Range	Main Muscle Groups	Type of Contraction	Minimum Ms Grade
ACTIVE rad/ul. joints.	$\sim\frac{1}{2}$	supinators pronators	conc/ecc. (vv) ecc/conc. (vv)	4 4
elbow	$\sim 90°$ flex	extensors flexors	concentric eccentric	4
shoulder	$\sim 45°$	flexors extensors adductors	concentric eccentric concentric	3+ 3
hand	gross grasp release	flexors extensors	concentric concentric	4 3
STATIC wrist				

Co-ordination

Gross Motor ■ control at shoulder, elbow, forearm and wrist;
■ accurate targeting and placement;
■ co-ordination between pronators and supinators.

Fine Motor ■ co-ordinated grasp/release to allow smooth action between supinators and pronators.

Gradation

	yes/no	How?
RESISTANCE	yes	alter stiffness of threads; alter material used (eg. plastic, metal).
RANGE OF MOTION	yes	start by using small movements, with many small turns; increase to larger movements and fewer turns.
CO-ORDINATION (gross/fine)	no	

Also used for:	How?
1 rad/ul. deviation	screwing action accomplished using rad/ul. deviation, forearm remains in pronation.
2 shoulder IR/ER	using straight arm, twisting action is accomplished using shoulder rotation.

Comments

When used for pronation/supination watch carefully that patient does not compensate by using shoulder rotation. Keep arm adducted.

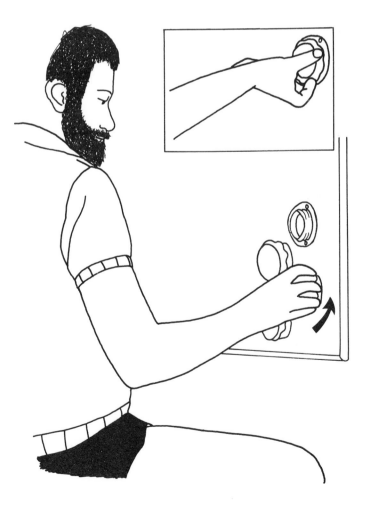

TITLE

Sheep (solitaire game)

MOVEMENT

Pronation and Supination

Category

Purposeful Activity, Light

Description

Patient sits at table with 'sheep board' in front of them. The board is set up with five red cylinders on one side, five white cylinders on the other and one vacant spot in the middle. The cylinders are to be transposed either by one move forward or by jumping over one cylinder – never go backwards.

To complete the game transpose the colours again to original set-up. The patient sits with arms at their side, elbows bent to 90°; grasp cylinders with palmar grasp, moving each cylinder by using pronation in one direction and supination in the other.

Equipment

▶ sheep board (~22″ long, 11 holes spaced 2″ apart), see illustration.

Skills required for activity as exercise
Action

Joints Used	Minimum Jt Range	Main Muscle Groups	Type of Contraction	Minimum Ms Grade
ACTIVE rad/ul. joints.	full	pronators supinators	conc/ecc. (vv) ecc/conc. (vv)	3+ 3+
hand	gross grasp	grasp/release	conc/ecc. (vv)	3+
shoulder	partial rotation and flex	rotators and flexors	conc/ecc. concentric	3+ 3+
STATIC elbow – flexed to 90° wrist				

Co-ordination

Gross Motor ■ control at shoulder and of pronation/supination.

Fine Motor ■ controlled sustained grasp and release;
■ accurate targeting and placement.

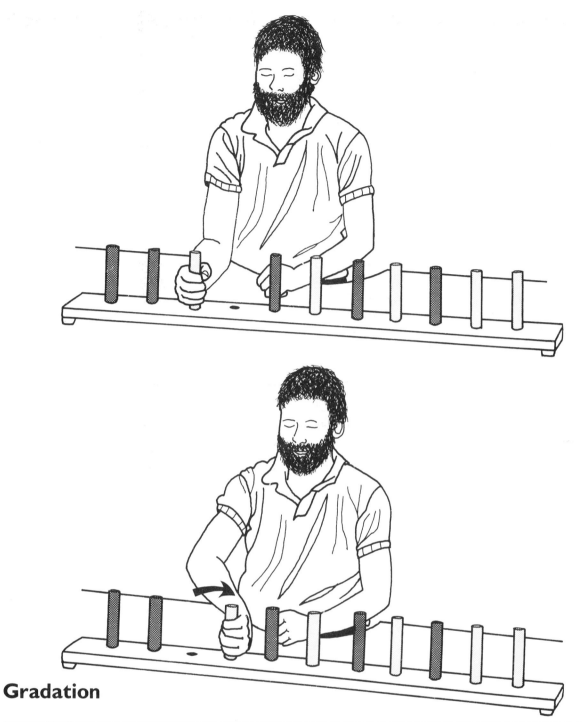

Gradation

	yes/no	How?
RESISTANCE	yes	alter weight of cylinders (eg. solid with varying weights to empty); can use velcro attachment to increase resistance.
RANGE OF MOTION	no	
CO-ORDINATION (gross/fine)	yes	alter size of cylinders to alter control required; for example, large velcro attachments would reduce control required.

Also used for:	How?
1 shoulder rotation	do with straight arms, using shoulder rotation to move cylinders.
2 elbow flex/ext.	use deeper holes and long dowels, lift dowels using elbow flexion.
3 shoulder flex/ext.	use dowels as sheep and move them using straight arms, lifting with shoulder flex.

Comments

Open cylinders can be used, starting with coloured water in each cylinder, except for one empty in the centre. To move, pour water into empty container and replace newly emptied container in original spot. Pouring action is done by using pronation/supination alternately. This requires more accurate motor control and incorporates a functional skill.

Alter shape, size, attachments, and so on as in methods of adapting solitaire.

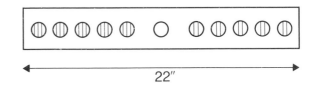

22"

TITLE
Table Football

MOVEMENT
Pronation/ Supination

Category

Purposeful Activity, Light

Equipment

▶ As figure below.

Description

Patient sits, arms at side, elbows bent to 90°; grasp handles of table football with forearms in mid-position. Move the ball around between 'players' by turning handles using pronation and supination alternately. The aim is to get the ball in the goal at the end. Can be played with two people and with more rows of players.

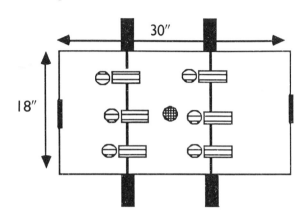

Skills required for activity as exercise
Action

Joints Used	Minimum Jt Range	Main Muscle Groups	Type of Contraction	Minimum Ms Grade
ACTIVE rad/ul. joints.	~¾	supinators pronators	conc/ecc. (vv) ecc/conc. (vv)	3+ 3+
hand	gross grasp	grasp	concentric	3+
STATIC elbow at ~90°				

Co-ordination

Gross Motor ■ co-ordination between supinators and pronators;
■ quick reactions, controlled targeting, good eye/hand co-ordination.

Fine Motor ■ sustained grasp.

Gradation

	yes/no	How?
RESISTANCE	yes	alter size and weight of ball (eg. polystyrene, hollow rubber, solid rubber, plastic).
RANGE OF MOTION	yes	work within available range from ¾ to full.
CO-ORDINATION (gross/fine)	yes	alter size of ball and target – smaller ball requires more control and quicker reactions.

Also used for:	How?
shoulder rotation	keep elbows straight, turn handles by using shoulder rotation.

MOVEMENT

Wrist Flexion

Prime Movers

Flexor Carpi Radialis

Flexor Carpi Ulnaris

Normal Range

0° to 90°

Nerve Supply

Medial ($C_{6,7}$)

Ulnar (C_8,T_1)

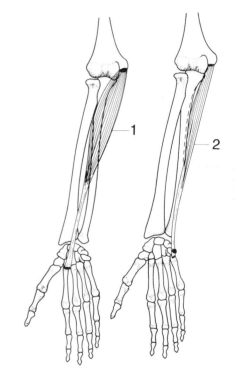

1 Flexor carpi radialis

2 Flexor carpi ulnaris

MOVEMENT

Wrist Extension

Prime Movers

Extensor Carpi Radialis Longus

Extensor Carpi Radialis Brevis

Extensor Carpi Ulnaris

Normal Range

0° to 70° (from mid-position)

Nerve Supply

Radial ($C_{6,7}$)

Radial ($C_{6,7}$)

Radial ($C_{6,7,8}$)

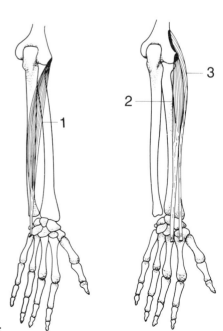

1 Extensor carpi ulnaris

2 Extensor carpi radialis brevis

3 Extensor carpi radialis longus

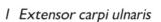

TITLE

Darts

MOVEMENT

Wrist Flexion/ Extension

Category

Purposeful Activity, Light

Description

Patient stands (or can sit if necessary) facing the dart board, a few feet away. Throw darts at the target using wrist extension to prepare and wrist flexion to throw. The elbow should only move about 45 degrees. The darts are held between the first two digits and thumb.

* See 'comments' below.

Equipment

▶ dart board mounted on an adjustable height wall bracket;
▶ darts.

Skills required for activity as exercise
Action

Joints Used	Minimum Jt Range	Main Muscle Groups	Type of Contraction	Minimum Ms Grade
ACTIVE wrist	$\sim\frac{1}{2}$	*Preparation:* extensors (release)	concentric	3+
		flexors	concentric	3+
		extensors	eccentric	
hand	full tripod pinch	pinch/release	conc/ecc (vv)	3+
elbow	$\sim45°$	flexors (prep)	concentric	3+
		extensors (rel)	concentric	3**
		flexors (rel)	eccentric	
STATIC shoulder at $\sim45°$				

Co-ordination

Gross Motor ■ control at shoulder, elbow, and wrist;
■ accurate targeting.

Fine Motor ■ controlled tripod pinch and release; timing essential;
■ good eye/hand co-ordination.

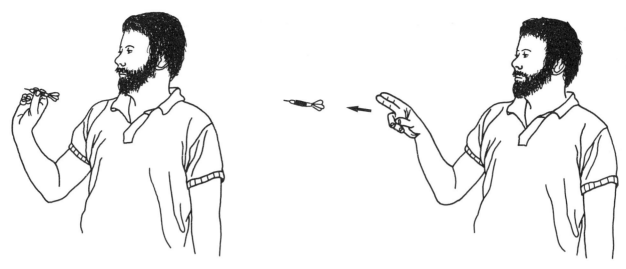

Gradation

	yes/no	How?
RESISTANCE	yes	alter size and weight of throwing objects (eg. use velcro target and polystyrene balls); alter distance from target.
RANGE OF MOTION	yes	alter distance from target; use available ROM but watch for over-compensation with elbow and shoulder.
CO-ORDINATION (gross/fine)	yes	alter by using larger target and larger throwing objects (as above); also this improves safety.

Also used for:	How?
elbow flex/ext.	throwing action done with elbow flex/ext; must increase standing distance from board.

Comments

* Gravity assists with elbow extension in this position; however for accurate, controlled release elbow flexors and extensors must work in a co-ordinated manner; grade 3+ is the minimum to allow for this control.

** Activity can also be done with patient in sitting position, forearm supported on a 'ski-jump' in pronation, with the target placed on the floor in front. The darts are thrown by bringing the wrist into extension for preparation and then releasing the dart as the wrist is brought down into flexion. This technique avoids compensatory movements at the elbow and shoulder.

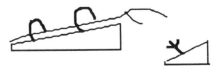

This is a potentially dangerous activity especially for those individuals lacking motor control and judgement. Patient must be carefully assessed and this activity only selected if appropriate.

TITLE ■■■■

Post Box

MOVEMENT ■■■■

Wrist Extension/ Flexion

Category

Purposeful Activity, Light

Description

Patient sits at table with forearm supported on an adjustable height 'ski jump' with forearm in pronation and stabilised with two dorsal, velcro attaching straps, one over the distal forearm and the other just distal to the elbow. Pick up objects placed in front of the platform and 'post' them through the holes in the upright board that is mounted a hand's width away from the 'ski jump'.

Reach down by flexing the wrist then bring the wrist up to 'post' objects using wrist extension.

Equipment

▶ 'ski jump' – type platform attached to the base by a hinge, to allow an adjustable angle; dorsal, velcro attaching straps at each end; all built into a wooden box with an upright board placed approx. $3\frac{1}{2}'' - 4''$ in front of the platform; the upright board has holes large enough for the placement of objects;

▶ objects, such as pegs, for 'posting'.

Skills required for activity as exercise
Action

Joints Used	Minimum Jt Range	Main Muscle Groups	Type of Contraction	Minimum Ms Grade
ACTIVE *Posting* wrist	$\sim\frac{1}{2}$	extensors	concentric	3+
hand	full tripod grasp	pinch/release	conc/ecc. (vv)	3+
Return to start wrist	full flex	flexors extensors	concentric eccentric	0 (gravity will assist) for controlled return

Co-ordination

Gross Motor ■ wrist control;
■ controlled repeated movement.

Fine Motor ■ controlled fine or tripod pinch and release at appropriate time;
■ accurated targeting and placement.

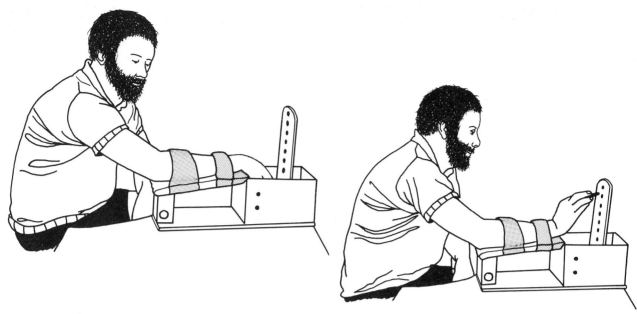

Gradation

	yes/no	How?
RESISTANCE	yes	alter weight of objects; add weights over dorsum of hand; use metal upright and metal underneath the 'ski jump' with magnetic attaching pieces.
RANGE OF MOTION	yes	build up bottom of box so patient does not have to use full wrist flex. to reach objects; alter by height of hole in which objects are placed (can number or colour levels for motivation).
CO-ORDINATION (gross/fine)	yes	alter size of objects and size of the hole in which they are placed.

Also used for:	How?
1 tenodesis training	pick up objects using wrist extension and passive tenodesis grasp, place objects on platform in front of hand rather than through the holes.
2 MCP and IP flex/ext.	same technique as for wrist flex/ext. with the emphasis on the finger movement.

Comments

Can be done using chair with elevated arm trough,
with upright board in front.

TITLE

'Ski Jump' With Weights

MOVEMENT

Wrist Flexion or Wrist Extension

Category

Therapeutic Exercise, Light to Moderate

Description

Patient sitting at table with arm supported on 'ski jump' and stabilised with velcro attaching strap just proximal to wrist.

Wrist Extension: forearm is pronated and sandbag weight placed over dorsal surface of hand; raise hand and weight with wrist extension.

Wrist Flexion: forearm is supinated and weight placed over palm; raise hand and weight by using wrist flexion.

Equipment

▶ 'ski jump' (*see Figure below*), adjustable angles if possible;

▶ varying weights, either sandbag or wrist cuffs.

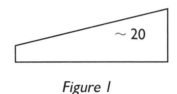

Figure 1

Skills required for activity as exercise
Action

Joints Used	Minimum Jt Range	Main Muscle Groups	Type of Contraction	Minimum Ms Grade
ACTIVE *Wrist Extension* wrist	$\sim\frac{1}{4}$	extensors flexors	concentric eccentric	3 (no wt.)
Wrist Flexion wrist	$\sim\frac{1}{4}$	flexors extensors	concentric eccentric	3 (no wt.)
STATIC elbow shoulder rad/ul.				

Co-ordination

Gross Motor ■ control at wrist;
    ■ controlled repetitive movement.

Fine Motor ■ none.

Gradation

	yes/no	How?
RESISTANCE	yes	alter weights, starting with gravity up to tolerated weight (5lb max.); with forearm resting on the ulnar border, do exercise with gravity eliminated.
RANGE OF MOTION	yes	can be done within available joint range.
CO-ORDINATION (gross/fine)	no	

Also used for:	How?
1 tenodesis training	same technique.
2 rad/ul. deviation	for rad. dev. forearm is supported on ulnar border and weight through web space;
	for ul. dev. forearm is supported on radial border and weight just proximal to 5th digit.
3 MCP flex/ext.	forearm and hand are supported to MCPs and weight placed just distal to MCPs.

Comments

When performing wrist extension, gravity may assist for return to starting position (wrist flexed). However, it is a more effective exercise if the patient makes a slow and controlled return to the starting position, thereby using an eccentric contraction of wrist extensors – an effective method of strengthening. This holds true for wrist flexion as well.

This can be made into a purposeful activity by incorporating a remedial game, done with the forearm supported on the 'ski jump' and the weights in the same position, but with a game in front of the 'ski jump'. This would require accurate fine motor control. It may provide more interest and therefore motivation for some individuals that have active, controlled hand function.

TITLE
Threaded Solitaire II

MOVEMENT
Wrist Flexion/ Extension

Category

Purposeful Activity, Light

Description

Patient stands facing the side of the mounted solitaire board. Patient plays solitaire by grasping the selected large threaded peg with a gross palmar grasp unscrewing it using wrist flexion and extension alternately, jumping, and screwing it into a vacant spot. Then remove the peg that was jumped by unscrewing it. The object is to end up with one peg left on the board.

Equipment

▶ large solitaire board with large pegs attached by threaded screws (see Figure 1);

▶ adjustable bracket for mounting.

Skills required for activity as exercise
Action

Joints Used	Minimum Jt Range	Main Muscle Groups	Type of Contraction	Minimum Ms Grade
ACTIVE *Unscrewing and Screwing* wrist	$\sim\frac{1}{2}$	extensors flexors	conc/ecc. ecc/conc.	3+–4 3+–4
hand	full gross grasp	grasp/release	conc/ecc. (vv)	4
shoulder	$\sim70°$	flexors	concentric	3+–4
STATIC elbow				

Co-ordination

Gross Motor ■ shoulder and wrist control.

Fine Motor ■ controlled grasp/release, coordinated with twisting action at wrist;
■ accurate targeting and placement to replace cylinders in threads.

Gradation

	yes/no	How?
RESISTANCE	yes	alter tightness of threads; alter weight of cylinders; alter material of cylinders (eg. plastic, wood, metal).
RANGE OF MOTION	yes	use small movements and many repetitions or larger movement and less repetitions.
CO-ORDINATION (gross/fine)	yes	alter target size (eg. smaller versus larger threads).

Also used for:	How?
1 rad/ul. deviation	face board, grasp cylinders (or other flatter screw in pieces) in palm, perform screwing action using rad/ul. deviation.
2 pron/sup.	face board, twist cylinders by using pron/sup.
3 MCP flex/ext.	use small pegs, grasp pegs at end of fingers and twist using alternate finger flex/ext.

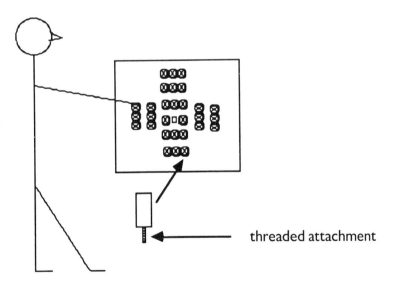

threaded attachment

Figure 1

MOVEMENT

MCP Flexion

Prime Movers

Third and Fourth Lumbricales

First and Second Lumbricales

Interossei Dorsales

Normal Range

0° to 90°

Range of motion

0° to 90°

Nerve Supply

Ulnar (C_8)

Median ($C_{6,7}$)

Ulnar (C_{8, T_1})

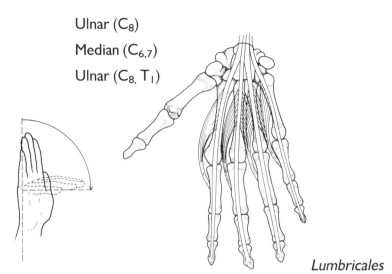

Lumbricales

MOVEMENT

MCP Extension

Prime Movers

Extensor Digitorum Communis

Extensor Indicis Proprius

Extensor Digiti Minimi

Normal Range

0° to 20° – 30°

Range of motion:

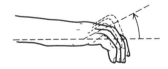

0° to 20° – 30°
Extension beyond
mid-line

Nerve Supply

Radial ($C_{6,7,8}$)

Radial ($C_{6,7,8}$)

Radial (C_7)

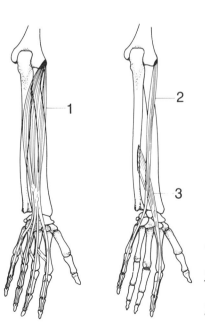

1 Extensor digitorum communis

2 Extensor digiti minimi

3 Extensor indicis proprius

TITLE
Bandage Roll

MOVEMENT
MCP Flexion/ Extension

Category

Therapeutic Exercise, Light

Equipment

▶ I crepe bandage.

Description

Patient sits at table with bandage stretched out on table. Roll bandage towards self keeping heel of hand on table and rolling with straight fingers, flexed only at the MCPs (*see Figure 1*). Can be done with both hands simultaneously.

Skills required for activity as exercise
Action

Joints Used	Minimum Jt Range	Main Muscle Groups	Type of Contraction	Minimum Ms Grade
ACTIVE *Rolling Action* MCPs	$\sim\frac{1}{2}$	intrinsics (lumbricals)	concentric	3+
wrist	$\sim\frac{1}{2}$ ext	extensors	concentric or isometric	3+
Returning to Starting Position MCPs	same	extensors	concentric	3
STATIC IPs				

Co-ordination

Gross Motor ■ proximal control for accurate hand function.

Fine Motor ■ can be done with two hands simultaneously, therefore requiring two-handed co-ordination;
■ repetitive, controlled straightening and flexing of MCPs.

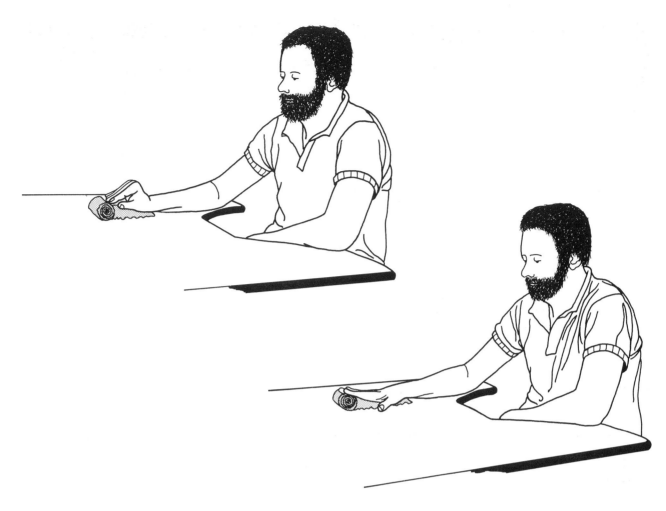

Figure 1

Gradation

	yes/no	How?
RESISTANCE	yes	alter rolling material; for example, use theraputty (*see Figure 2*), playdough, towel or just do pure movement initially along table (use powder to decrease resistance).
RANGE OF MOTION	yes	can work within available range starting from approximately half.
CO-ORDINATION (gross/fine)	no	

Also used for:	How?
IP flex/ext.	rolling action done with IP flexion.

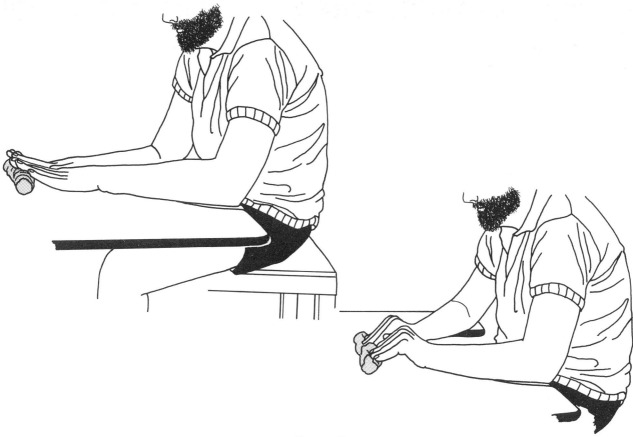

Figure 2

TITLE

Finger Extension Game

MOVEMENT

MCP Flexion/ Extension

Category

Purposeful Activity, Light

Equipment

▶ ping pong balls of varying weights from 0 to 0.225kg ($\frac{1}{2}$ lb).

Description

Patient sits with forearm supported and strapped into pronation on 'ski jump' with only fingers protruding over edge. Place ball in one of the three dimples in front of the relaxed fingers. The backboard is placed at one of the three positions appropriate to the patient's strength. Patient flicks ball at one of the four targets using MCP extension, alternating fingers. Targets are numbered and score can be kept.

Skills required for activity as exercise
Action

Joints Used	Minimum Jt Range	Main Muscle Groups	Type of Contraction	Minimum Ms Grade
ACTIVE *Preparation* MCPs	~$\frac{3}{4}$ flex.	intrinsics	concentric	3—
Flicking MCPs	~$\frac{1}{4}$	extensors intrinsics flexors	concentric concentric eccentric	3 3
STATIC IPs wrist				

Co-ordination

Gross Motor ■ none except sitting balance.

Fine Motor ■ accurate control of MCP extension for flicking action;
■ accurate targeting (although not mandatory if targets not used).

Gradation

	yes/no	How?
RESISTANCE	yes	alter weight of ping pong balls; alter distance of target.
RANGE OF MOTION	yes	can be done within available range; alter distance of target.
CO-ORDINATION (gross/fine)	yes	alter size of balls – smaller balls (eg. marbles) require finer control and accuracy than larger (eg. ping pong balls).

Also used for:	How?
1 IP extension	support hand to the PIPs and then DIPs, (then must lower support wedge).
2 wrist extension	adjust height of wedge, support forearm to wrist, use wrist extension for flicking action.

Comments

To return hand to starting position wrist can be dropped; therefore active MCP flexion is not absolutely essential to complete the activity.

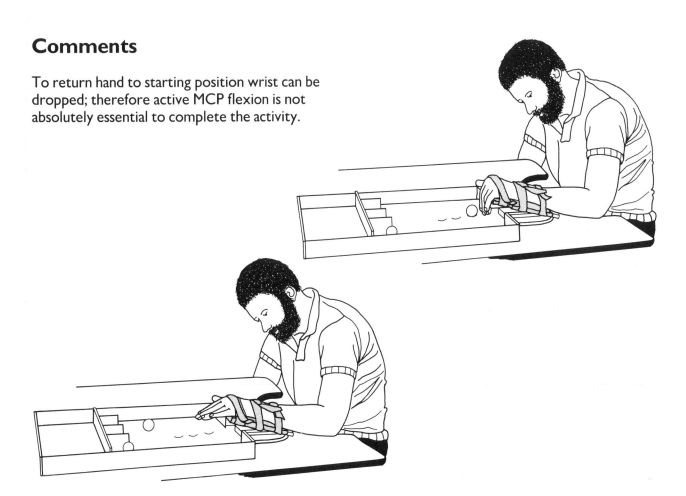

TITLE
Lumbrical Box Game

MOVEMENT
MCP Flexion/ Extension

Category

Therapeutic Exercise, Light

Description

Half fill the lumbrical box (see *Equipment* for description) with marbles. A lid with an oval cut out is placed on top. The patient picks out as many marbles as possible from the box. The patient can compete against the clock or another person.

Equipment

▶ a small wooden box, 5″ square with a lid with an oval cut-out just large enough to allow the thumb and fingers to fit through if fingers are straight;

▶ marbles to half fill the box.

Skills required for activity as exercise
Action

Joints Used	Minimum Jt Range	Main Muscle Groups	Type of Contraction	Minimum Ms Grade
ACTIVE *Grasp* MCPs	full flex	intrinsics (esp. lumbricals)	concentric	3+
thumb	full	flexors adductor	concentric concentric	3+ 3+
Release MCPs	$\sim\frac{1}{4}$ ext.	extensors	concentric	3−
thumb	$\sim\frac{1}{4}$ ext.	extensors abductor	concentric concentric	2 2
STATIC IPs wrist				

Co-ordination

Gross Motor ■ proximal control required for accurate hand function.

Fine Motor ■ controlled grasp/release with fingers straight;
■ sustained grasp.

Gradation

	yes/no	How?
RESISTANCE	yes	alter weight of objects being picked up (eg. polystyrene balls, lead ball-bearings).
RANGE OF MOTION	yes	alter size of objects being picked up (eg. ping pong balls, small ball-bearings).
CO-ORDINATION (gross/fine)	no	

Also used for:	How?
see *interossei box* game	

Comments

Vision is occluded by lid and therefore it is mandatory that the patient have intact sensation to light touch and stereognosis.

Alternatively the front of the box may be made with plexiglass so the patient can see objects to be picked up and can watch that movement is being done correctly.

To incorporate into a sensory exercise as well, fill box with various materials such as sand, rice, oatmeal, polystyrene chips and so on and have patient find the objects in that.

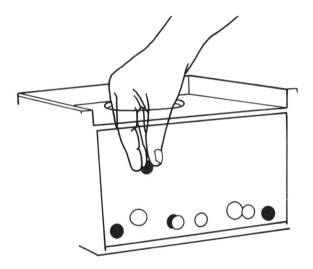

TITLE
Lumbrical Sanding

MOVEMENT
MCP Flexion

Category

Therapeutic Exercise, Purposeful Activity, Moderate

Description

Patient standing or sitting with piece of wood and sander in front of them. Strap hand into sander with fingers straight and flexed at the MCPs. Sand piece of wood. Can be incorporated into project if appropriate.

Equipment

► wooden block shaped into a peak (*see Figure 1*) with sandpaper on the bottom and a velcro attaching strap to go over the PIPs.

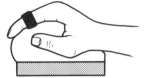

Skills required for activity as exercise
Action

Joints Used	Minimum Jt Range	Main Muscle Groups	Type of Contraction	Minimum Ms Grade
ACTIVE MCPs	$\sim\frac{1}{2}$	intrinsics	isometric	3+
wrist	$\sim\frac{1}{2}$	extensors	isometric	3+–4
shoulder or elbow	$\sim\frac{1}{2}$	horiz. add/abd flex/ext.	conc/ecc. (vv) conc/ecc. (vv)	3+ 3+
STATIC IPs thumb				

Co-ordination

Gross Motor ■ shoulder and elbow control required.

Fine Motor ■ no fine motor control required as hand is fixed in sander. However, if incorporated into project involving small parts, accurate fine control may be required.

Gradation

	yes/no	How?
RESISTANCE	yes	harder or softer wolds could be used to increase or decrease resistance. Different grades of sandpaper could also be used to achieve the same effect. Resistance can be reduced by using the block and a polisher and replacing the sandpaper with a padded cloth.
RANGE OF MOTION	yes	alter angle of peak on sander.
CO-ORDINATION (gross/fine)	yes	alter size and complexity of object to be sanded.

Also used for:	How?
1 shoulder 2 elbow 3 wrist	see 'Sanding' under *Shoulder Flexion*.

Comments

Lumbrical sanders are commercially available.

TITLE
Sponge Ball Squeeze

MOVEMENT
MCP Flexion/ Extension

Category

Therapeutic Exercise, Moderate

Equipment

▶ one bowl of warm water and one empty bowl; various sizes and densities of sponge balls.

Description

Start with sponge balls of various sizes in a bowl of water. Ask patient to take them one at a time and squeeze them dry into the adjacent empty bowl, the object being to empty one bowl of water into the other. The squeezing action is accomplished by placing the sponge ball between the thumb and straight fingers and squeezing them together, keeping fingers straight throughout the exercise.

Skills required for activity as exercise
Action

Joints Used	Minimum Jt Range	Main Muscle Groups	Type of Contraction	Minimum Ms Grade
ACTIVE *Squeeze* MCPs	$\sim\frac{3}{4}$	intrinsics extensors	concentric eccentric	4
thumb	$\sim\frac{3}{4}$	flexors adductor	concentric concentric	4 4
Release * MCPs	same	extensors	concentric	3−
thumb	same	extensors abductors	concentric concentric	2 2

Co-ordination

Gross Motor ■ trunk stability required for sitting balance.

Fine Motor ■ repeated sustained grasp (with extended fingers) and controlled release.

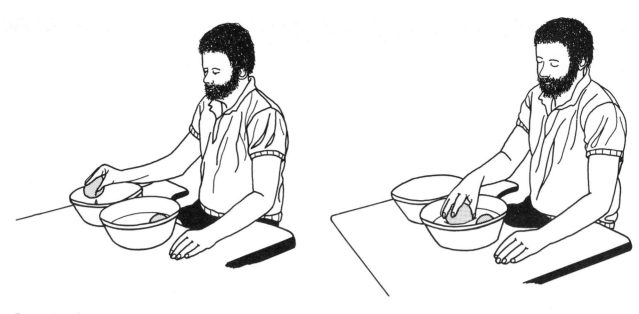

Gradation

	yes/no	How?
RESISTANCE	yes	alter density of sponge; for reduced resistance movement can be made without sponge by flexing at MCPs with IPs straight – either by free-floating or by moving fingers along bottom of bowl with heel of hand resting on bottom.
RANGE OF MOTION	yes	alter size of sponge (larger sponges require less range).
CO-ORDINATION (gross/fine)	no	

Also used for:	How?
1 wrist flex/ext. (tenodesis training)	support wrist on 'ski jump' with bowl of water in front and below hand, reach for sponge ball with wrist flexion and bring up and squeeze with wrist extension.
2 IP flexion	hold and squeeze ball in palm using IP flexion to squeeze water out.
3 grasp strengthening	squeeze ball using gross grasp.
4 pinch	squeeze ball using pinch between thumb and each finger alternately.

Comments

* Release can be achieved by dropping wrist, in which case active use of finger and thumb extensors would be unnecessary.

■

TITLE

T–Shaped Solitaire

MOVEMENT

MCP Extension/ Flexion

Category

Purposeful Activity, Moderate

Description

Patient sits at table with forearm supported in pronation on 'ski jump', solitaire board with velcro attached, T-shaped pieces immediately in front of hand. The patient plays solitaire by holding the pieces between two fingers, just distal to the MCPs and lifts to remove, using MCP extension.

Equipment

▶ solitaire board with T-shaped pieces attached to board with either velcro or pegs;

▶ 'ski jump'.

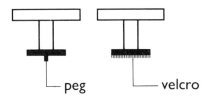

Skills required for activity as exercise
Action

Joints Used	Minimum Jt Range	Main Muscle Groups	Type of Contraction	Minimum Ms Grade
ACTIVE *Removing* MCPs	$\sim\frac{1}{2}$	extensors flexors intrinsics (esp. interossei)	concentric eccentric concentric	4 4
wrist * *Replacing* MCPs	same	interossei extensors flexors	concentric isometric isometric	3+

Co-ordination

Gross Motor ■ proximal control required for accurate hand function.

Fine Motor ■ accurate control of intrinsics and long extensors;
■ repetitive, controlled grasp/ release between fingers.

Gradation

	yes/no	How?
RESISTANCE	yes	alter method of attachment (eg. use peg attachments to decrease resistance).
RANGE OF MOTION	no	
CO-ORDINATION (gross/fine)	no	

Also used for:	How?
IP extension	hold pieces between fingers, immediately distal to the PIPs, lift by straightening fingers.

Comments

* Some wrist action may come in, but it is important to watch that MCP extension is not compromised by this. It may be necessary for the patient to stabilise their wrist with the other hand.

TITLE

Tong Solitaire

MOVEMENT

MCP Flexion/ Extension

Category

Purposeful Activity, Light

Description

Patient sits at table with Solitaire game in front of them. Have patient pick up, move and remove pegs, holding and squeezing tongs between thumb and straight fingers. To play the game every hole on the board but one is filled. Move by jumping one peg over one other into a vacant spot. Remove the peg that was jumped. The object is to leave one peg on the board – preferably in the spot that was originally vacant. Hold tongs between thumb and alternate fingers.

Equipment

▶ braintease board (approx. 10″ × 10″ × 10″), pegs;

▶ tongs (wooden or kitchen) and elastic bands.

This can also be done with 'bulldog clips', car battery clamps, large or small kitchen or barbecue tongs.

Skills required for activity as exercise
Action

Joints Used	Minimum Jt Range	Main Muscle Groups	Type of Contraction	Minimum Ms Grade
ACTIVE *Close* MCPs	$\sim\frac{1}{2}-\frac{3}{4}$	flexors intrinsics extensors	concentric concentric eccentric	3+ 3+
thumb	$\sim\frac{1}{2}$	flexors adductor extensors	concentric concentric eccentric	3+ 3+
Open MCPs	same	extensors flex/intrinsics	concentric eccentric	3
thumb	same	extensors abductors flexors	concentric concentric eccentric	3 3

Co-ordination

Gross Motor ■ proximal control for accurate hand function.

Fine Motor ■ accurate targeting and placement;

■ controlled open/close;

■ good eye/hand co-ordination.

Gradation

	yes/no	How?
RESISTANCE	yes	place elastic bands around the end of the tongs, alter tension of tongs used; on some tongs position of grip on handle can alter tension (more difficult when held at top); can be done without tongs, just using fingers to hold and move pegs.
RANGE OF MOTION	yes	alter size of pegs.
CO-ORDINATION (gross/fine)	yes	alter size of pegs – larger pegs require less fine motor control.

Also used for:	How?
1 pinch	use tweezers instead of tongs; hold tweezers between thumb and distal end of alternate fingers.
2 IP flexion	as for pinch, or patient can pick up pegs without tweezers, just between thumb and distal end of fingers.

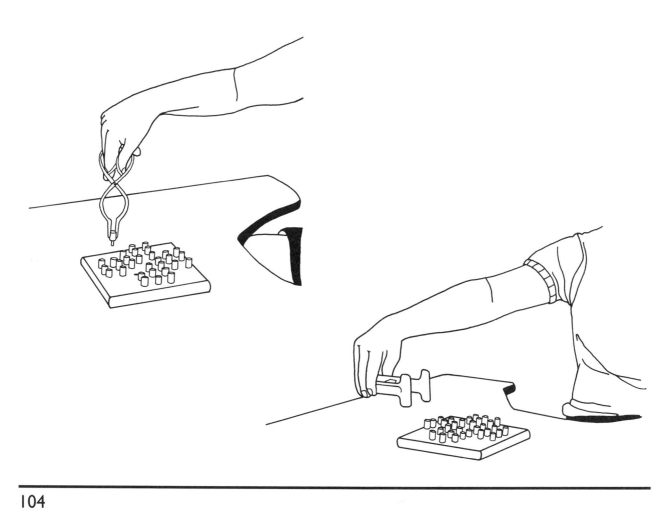

MOVEMENT

Finger Abduction

Prime Movers

Interossei Dorsales

Abductor Digiti Minimi

Nerve Supply

Ulnar (C_8, T_1)

Ulnar (C_8)

Normal Range

$0°$ to $20° - 25°$

Range of motion:

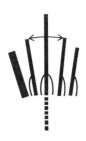

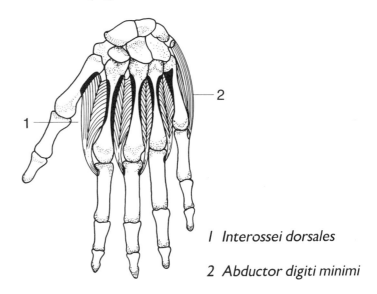

1 *Interossei dorsales*

2 *Abductor digiti minimi*

MOVEMENT

Finger Adduction

Prime Movers

Interossei Palmares

Nerve Supply

Ulnar (C_8, T_1)

Normal Range

$20° - 25°$ to $0°$

Range of motion:

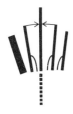

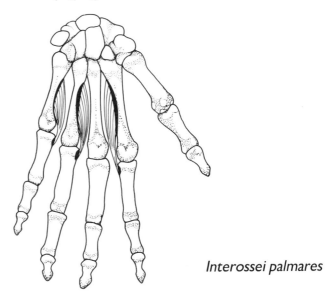

Interossei palmares

TITLE ▮▮▮▮▮▮▮

| Coin Travel |

MOVEMENT ▮▮▮▮▮▮▮

| Finger Abduction/ Adduction |

Category

Therapeutic Exercise, Light

Equipment

▶ coins of various sizes, from 1p to 50p.

Description

Have patient hold coin between thumb and index finger. With heel of hand or wrist resting on table-top move the coin over fingers to between fourth and fifth digits and back again. The patient can race the clock or another person if appropriate.

Skills required for activity as exercise
Action

Joints Used	Minimum Jt. Range	Main Muscle Groups	Type of Contraction	Minimum Ms. Grade
ACTIVE MCPs	full	intrinsics flexors extensors	concentric conc/ecc. ecc/conc.	3+–4 3 3
STATIC wrist				

Co-ordination

Gross Motor ■ proximal control for accurate hand function.

Fine Motor ■ good fine motor co-ordination required.

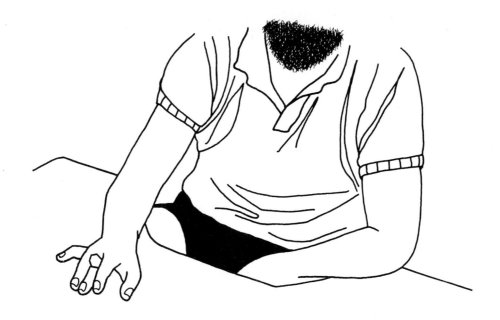

Gradation

	yes/no	How?
RESISTANCE	yes	can use masking tape; start at index finger and ask patient to move it to fifth digit; this requires slightly less strength than with coins.
RANGE OF MOTION	yes	alter size of coin – larger coins require slightly less ROM; can also be done by rolling pencils of various lengths between fingers.
CO-ORDINATION (gross/fine)	no	a high degree of co-ordination is required.

Comments

This exercise is only appropriate for late stages of rehabilitation.

TITLE
Interossei Box

MOVEMENT
Finger Adduction/Abduction

Category

Therapeutic Exercise, Light

Description

Half fill the interossei box (see description under *Equipment*) with marbles. The opening in the lid is too narrow to allow the thumb to enter. The patient picks out as many marbles as possible by using finger adduction. Can be played against the clock or another individual.

Equipment

▶ a small wooden box, 5″ square, with a lid that has an oval cut out that is too narrow to allow the thumb to enter, but allows all the fingers (perhaps use the same box as for *Lumbrical Game,* with different lid);

▶ marbles to half fill the box.

Skills required for activity as exercise
Action

Joints Used	Minimum Jt Range	Main Muscle Groups	Type of Contraction	Minimum Ms Grade
ACTIVE *Grasp* MCPs	full	intrinsics (interossei)	conc/ecc.	3+
Release MCPs		intrinsics (interossei)	conc/ecc.	2
STATIC IPs wrist				

Co-ordination

Gross Motor ■ proximal control for accurate hand function.

Fine Motor ■ controlled grasp/release between fingers;
■ sustained finger grasp.

Gradation

	yes/no	How?
RESISTANCE	yes	alter weight of objects to be picked up (eg. polystyrene, lead ball-bearings).
RANGE OF MOTION	yes	alter size of objects to be picked up – this is somewhat limited by the size of the box opening.
CO-ORDINATION (gross/fine)	no	

Comments

Because vision is occluded by lid, sensation to light touch and intact stereognosis are mandatory.

Alternatively, put a plexiglass front on the box so that:
(a) patient can use vision to see objects to be picked up – therefore intact sensation is not required;
(b) patient and therapist can watch that movement is being carried out correctly.

A sensory activity can also be incorporated by filling the box with various materials such as rice, oatmeal, sand or polystyrene chips. Place various objects in the material and ask the patient to find them using finger add/abduction to bring them out of the box.

TITLE

Interossei Sheep

MOVEMENT

Finger Adduction/ Abduction

Category

Purposeful Activity, Light

Equipment

▶ board about 12″ long with 9 holes for $\sim\frac{1}{2}''$ pegs;

▶ 4 white pegs, 4 black pegs.

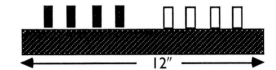

Description

Use a board as shown in illustration with four white pegs at one end and four black pegs at the other, with the centre hole open. The object is to reverse the position of the black and white pegs by moving one peg at a time, either to a single adjacent spot or to jump over an adjacent peg into an empty space. White can only be moved in one direction and black the other. To move the pegs, hold them between alternate fingers, keeping fingers straight (using interossei muscles).

Skills required for activity as exercise
Action

Joints Used	Minimum Jt. Range	Main Muscle Groups	Type of Contraction	Minimum Ms. Grade
ACTIVE *Hold & Release* MCPs Involvement of shoulder, elbow or wrist for movement along board	$\sim\frac{1}{2}$	intrinsics (interossei)	concentric and eccentric	3+ 2 for release

Co-ordination

Gross Motor ■ requires proximal control for accurate hand control and placement of pegs.

Fine Motor ■ accurate targeting and placement;
■ controlled grasp/release between fingers.

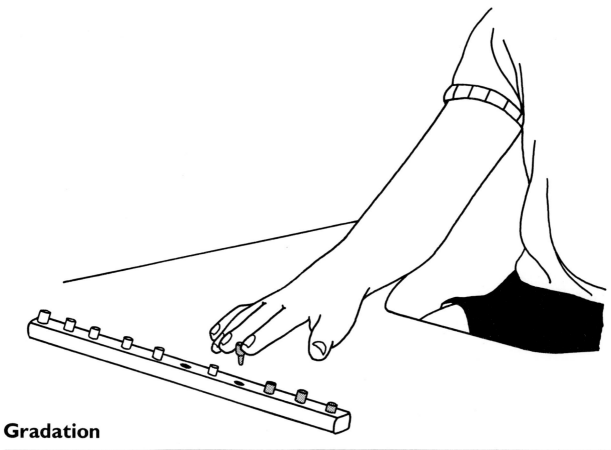

Gradation

	yes/no	How?
RESISTANCE	yes	alter weight of pegs (eg. polystyrene, plastic, wood, lead); to increase resistance adapt board with velcro attachment and put velcro on bottom of pegs.
RANGE OF MOTION	yes	alter size of pegs – thinner pegs require more range.
CO-ORDINATION (gross/fine)	yes	alter size of pegs – thinner pegs require more control for placement.

Also used for:	How?
1 pinch	pick up pegs using pinch with alternate fingers.
2 IP flex	as for pinch.

Comments

Other goals may be incorporated into this game by placing it at varying heights and angles (for example, incorporate shoulder flexion by placing it in front of the patient at shoulder level).

TITLE

Tug O' War II

MOVEMENT

Finger Abduction/ Adduction

Category

Purposeful Activity, Moderate

Description

Have patient hold one end of paper between any two fingers (alternate each time), keeping MCPs extended. Grasp the other end between the same two fingers of the other hand. Pull equally in

opposite directions: that is, have a tug of war with yourself. Can also be done between two people (eg. patient and therapist or two patients).

Equipment

▶ paper.

Skills required for activity as exercise
Action

Joints Used	Minimum Jt Range	Main Muscle Groups	Type of Contraction	Minimum Ms Grade
ACTIVE MCPs	full	intrinsics flexors extensors	concentric isometric isometric	3+–4
STATIC IPs wrist				

Co-ordination

Gross Motor ■ proximal control for accurate hand function.

Fine Motor ■ sustained closure of fingers;
■ ability to co-ordinate two arms working in opposition simultaneously (this is not necessary if opposed to another person).

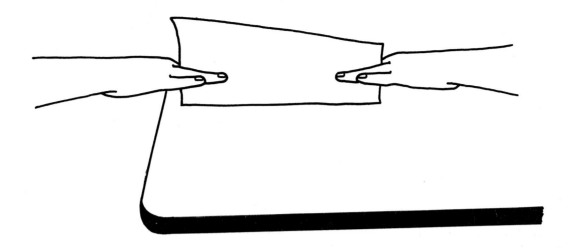

Gradation

	yes/no	How?
RESISTANCE	yes	alter resistance by amount of pull provided by other hand or opponent; can also be done with theraputty, squeezing it between fingers and pulling apart.
RANGE OF MOTION	yes	alter thickness of object for pulling (eg. use a cloth, small towel).
CO-ORDINATION (gross/fine)	yes	decreased co-ordination required if done against another person rather than self.

MOVEMENT

IP Flexion

Prime Movers

Flexor Digitorum Superficialis

Flexor Digitorum Profundus

Normal Range

PIPs: 0° to 120°

DIPs: 0° to 80°

Range of motion:

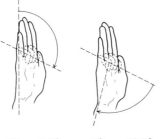

0° to 80°   0° to 120°

Nerve Supply

Median ($C_{7,8}$,T_1)

Ulnar (C_8,T_1)

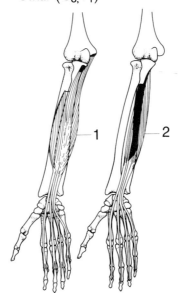

1 *Flexor digitorum superficialis*

2 *Flexor digitorum profundas*

MOVEMENT

IP Extension

Prime Movers

Extensor Digitorum Communis

Extensor Indicis Proprius

Extensor Digiti Minimi

Normal Range

PIPs: 120° to 0°

DIPS: 80° to 0°

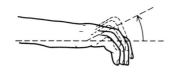

Nerve Supply

Radial ($C_{6,7,8}$)

Radial ($C_{6,7,8}$)

Radial (C_7)

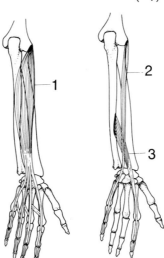

Dorsal View of Forearm and Hand

1 *Extensor digitorum communis*

2 *Extensor digiti minimi*

3 *Extensor indicis proprius*

TITLE ■■■■■■
Nuts and Bolts

MOVEMENT ■■■■■
IP Flexion

Category

Therapeutic Exercise, Moderate

Equipment

▶ bolts of various sizes in wooden frame, as shown in illustration;

▶ stop-watch (if appropriate).

Description

With nuts and bolts mounted as shown in *Figure 1* ask patient to unscrew all the nuts from one side and then screw them onto the bolts of the other side. This can be done by placing the nut between the thumb and any finger(s). Time if appropriate.

Skills required for activity as exercise
Action

Joints Used	Minimum Jt Range	Main Muscle Groups	Type of Contraction	Minimum Ms Grade
ACTIVE MCPs IPs	approx. $\frac{1}{2}$	*Screwing* * flexors intrinsics	concentric concentric	3+ 3+
		Unscrewing extensors intrinsics	concentric eccentric	3+
STATIC thumb wrist				

Co-ordination

Gross Motor ■ proximal control required.

Fine Motor ■ accurate control flexors/ extensors in rhythm;
■ co-ordinated grasp/release at IPs.

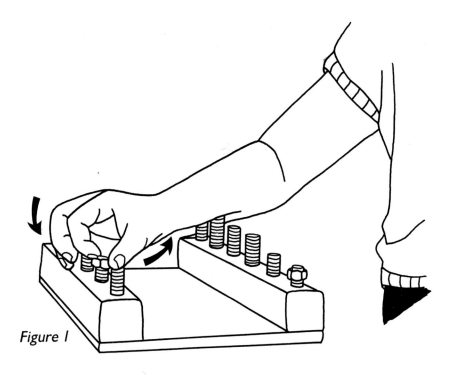

Figure 1

Gradation

	yes/no	How?
RESISTANCE	yes	alter the tension or size of the nuts and bolts used.
RANGE OF MOTION	yes	alter size of nuts and bolts.
CO-ORDINATION (gross/fine)	yes	use larger nuts and bolts for less control and smaller ones for more control.

Also used for:	How?
pinch strengthening and dexterity	same technique.

Comments

* The muscle groups listed are for the screwing action. After each flexion movement, it is necessary to open the hand slightly in order to replace the fingers for the next screwing action. The muscles required for opening are not listed specifically but are the same as those required for the unscrewing action.

This activity can be timed, comparing the left and right hands and/or one can compare between sessions.

TITLE ■■■■
Beads

MOVEMENT ■■■■
IP Flexion/Extension

Category

Purposeful Activity, Light

Description

Patient holds first bead in one hand and threading material (string, leather, wire, plastic) in the other. Thread material through hole of bead. Repeat until threading material is filled with beads. Hold beads and thread between thumb and alternate fingers.

Equipment

▶ threading material (eg. string, leather, wire, plastic, shoe lace)

▶ beads of various sizes.

Skills required for activity as exercise
Action

Joints Used	Minimum Jt Range	Main Muscle Groups	Type of Contraction	Minimum Ms Grade
ACTIVE *Grasping and Threading* MCPs/IPs	$\sim\frac{1}{2}$	flexors intrinsics	concentric concentric	3 2–3
thumb	$\sim\frac{1}{2}$	flexors	concentric	3
Releasing Beads MCPs/IPs	same	extensors	concentric	3–
STATIC wrist				

Co-ordination

Gross Motor ■ proximal control required for accurate hand function.

Fine Motor ■ accurate target and placement;
■ good eye/hand co-ordination;
■ controlled grasp/release;
■ ability to perform two-handed activity, both hands acting separately simultaneously.

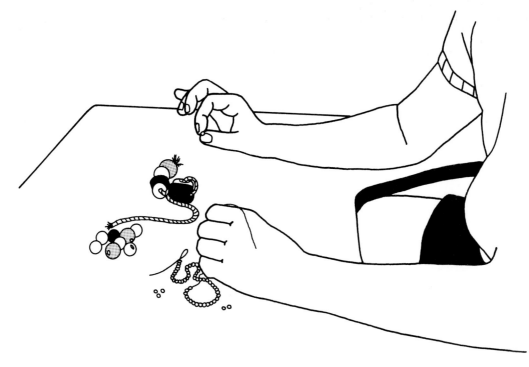

Gradation

	yes/no	How?
RESISTANCE	yes	alter weight of beads used (eg. polystyrene, plastic, wooden).
RANGE OF MOTION	yes	alter size of beads used.
CO-ORDINATION (gross/fine)	yes	to increase or decrease motor control requirements, alter size of beads and/or thickness and stiffness of threading material.

Also used for:	How?
1 Pinch strengthening and dexterity	same technique.
2 MCP flex/ext.	for lumbricals, hold beads and threading material with straight fingers using only MCP flexion.

Comments

For increased interest (and perhaps perceptual work) use various coloured beads and provide pattern cards to follow.

This activity also incorporates some forearm pronation and supination.

TITLE ∎
Elastics

MOVEMENT ∎
IP Extension

Category

Therapeutic Exercise, Moderate

Description

Five techniques:

1) 'Ski jump' with elastics or theraband on the front surface (*see Figure 1*).
2) Elastic design board (*see Figure 2*).
3) Plain elastics or theraband around fingers and thumb (*see Figure 3*). Extend IPs, stretching elastic outwards.

4) Attach two elastics; place one around the wrist holding forearm in supination. Bring second elastic up from centre of wrist to the appropriate finger. Straighten out finger, stretching the elastic back (*see Figure 4*).
5) Use various sizes of disks attached to a cylinder. Stretch elastics over the disk and place on the cylinder (*see Figure 5*).

Equipment

▶ See illustrations.

Skills required for activity as exercise
Action

Joints Used	Minimum Jt Range	Main Muscle Groups	Type of Contraction	Minimum Ms Grade
(Depends on elastic activity chosen) ACTIVE IPs	~30°	flexors/extensors	conc/ecc. (vv)	4
STATIC MCPs wrist				

Co-ordination

Gross Motor ∎ no gross motor control required except for trunk stability for sitting; some elastic exercise can be done lying down.

Fine Motor ∎ controlled opening and closing of fingers.

Gradation

	yes/no	How?
RESISTANCE	yes	alter tension of theraband or elastic bands used.
RANGE OF MOTION	yes	can be done within available range from 30°.
CO-ORDINATION (gross/fine)	no	

Also used for:	How?
MCP extension	support hand to MCPs, press into theraband using MCP extension; or place elastic just proximal to PIP.

Comments

Can be done like weight-lifting programme, counting repetitions and recording after each treatment session.

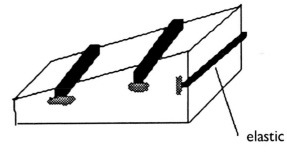

elastic

Figure 1

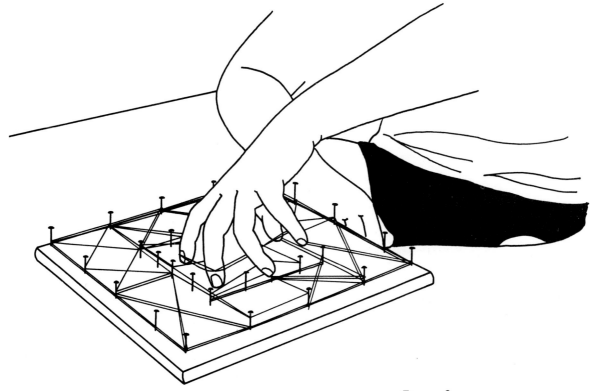

Figure 2

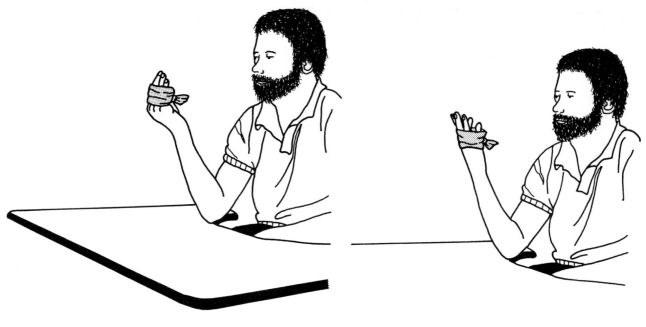

Figure 3

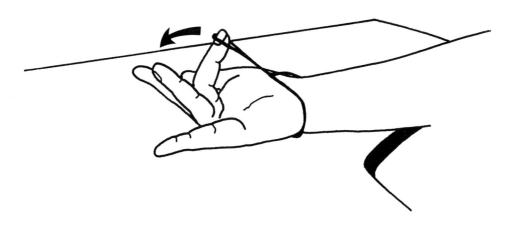

Figure 4

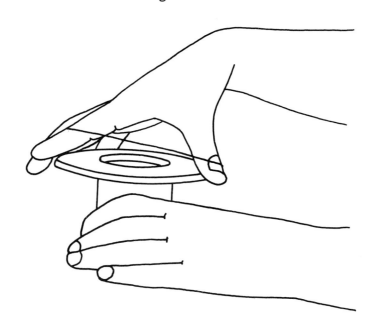

Figure 5

Category

Therapeutic Exercise, Moderate

Equipment

▶ theraputty of varying densities (resistance);

▶ table top.

Description

Using 'theraputty' flattened on table in front of seated patient, place hand palm-down on putty with IP joints in flexion. Push putty forward and out while straightening IP joints; bend IPs again and repeat.

Skills required for activity as exercise
Action

Joints Used	Minimum Jt Range	Main Muscle Groups	Type of Contraction	Minimum Ms Grade
ACTIVE IPs	$\frac{1}{4}$	intrinsics extensors flexors	concentric concentric eccentric	3+ 3+
STATIC MCPs (in neutral) wrist				

Co-ordination

Gross Motor ■ proximal stability.

Fine Motor ■ controlled opening and closing of fingers;
■ fine control demands are minimal.

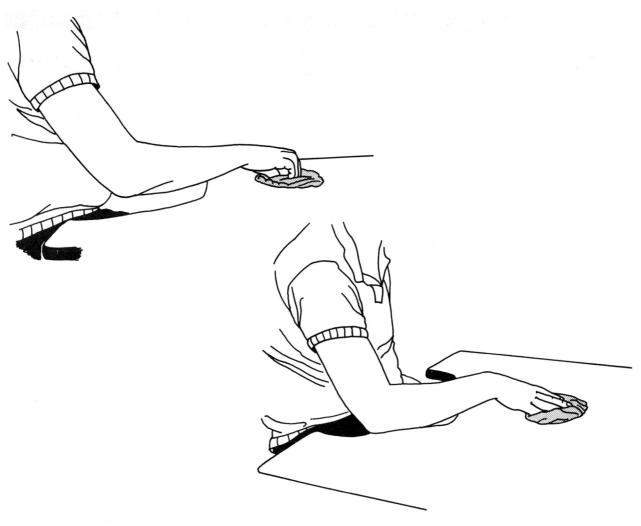

Gradation

	yes/no	How?
RESISTANCE	yes	can be done on table surface without putty; use baby powder to further decrease resistance; also use tissue to push out; alter density of putty.
RANGE OF MOTION	yes	can be done within available range from $\sim\frac{1}{4}$.
CO-ORDINATION (gross/fine)	no	

Also used for:	How?
1 MCP extension	start with fingers bent at the MCPs, push putty out by straightening whole finger from MCPs.
2 MCP/IP flexion	pull pancake in towards the centre using finger flexion.

TITLE

Pin Solitaire

MOVEMENT

IP Flexion/Extension

Category

Purposeful Activity, Light

Description

Using a polystyrene board with fine pins set up in solitaire formation with an empty space in the centre. Grasp a pin with fine pinch and jump over an adjoining pin to an empty space beyond, then remove the pin that was jumped. Pins may only be moved horizontally or vertically. The objective is to end up with one pin in the centre. Pins are moved by pinching them between the thumb and tip of each finger alternately.

Equipment

▶ polystyrene-covered board, approx. 8″ × 8″ (20cm × 20cm);

▶ pins.

Skills required for activity as exercise
Action

Joints Used	Minimum Jt Range	Main Muscle Groups	Type of Contraction	Minimum Ms Grade
ACTIVE *Grasp* IPs	~80°	finger flexors IP extensors	concentric eccentric	3+
thumb	a few degrees	flexors extensors	concentric eccentric	3+
Release * IPs		extensors	concentric	3−
thumb		extensors	concentric	2
STATIC wrist				

Co-ordination

Gross Motor ■ proximal control.

Fine Motor ■ accurate targeting and placement;
■ controlled pinch/release.

Gradation

	yes/no	How?
RESISTANCE	yes	alter density of polystyrene or foam in which the pins are placed; use fine tweezers to pick up pins.
RANGE OF MOTION	yes	alter size of pin head (eg. pad with foam or use pins with ball tops).
CO-ORDINATION (gross/fine)	no	

Also used for:	How?
1 fine pinch	same technique.
2 MCP flexion	for lumbricals, pick up pins with straight fingers.

Comments

* If active finger extension is weak or non-existent, release by dropping wrist. For controlled release minimum of grade 3– is required.

For individuals with altered sensation, be careful using pins – often even the top is quite sharp, especially when pushing into polystyrene.

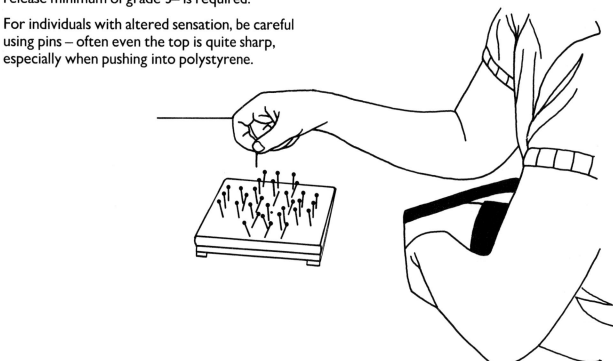

TITLE

Fluid Pump

MOVEMENT

Grasp Strengthening

Category

Therapeutic Exercise, Moderate

Description

Hold bulb in palm of hand, squeeze it hard, maintaining the grasp while the water travels from one flask to another. Hold to the count of five and then release. Repeat until the desired amount of fluid has been transferred to the other container.

Equipment

▶ two flasks each half-filled with coloured water;

▶ clear tubing with rubber bulb attached to the end, tubing inserted into one flask;

▶ another clear tube between flasks (for passage of fluid).

Skills required for activity as exercise
Action

Joints Used	Minimum Jt Range	Main Muscle Groups	Type of Contraction	Minimum Ms Grade
ACTIVE *Grasp* MCPs/IPs thumb	$\sim\frac{3}{4}$ $\sim\frac{3}{4}$	flexors flexors	concentric concentric	3+–4 3+–4
Release MCPs/IPs thumb	as above as above	extensors extensors	concentric concentric	3– 2
STATIC wrist				

Co-ordination

Gross Motor ■ none required except for trunk stability for sitting or standing.

Fine Motor ■ controlled grasp/release;
■ sustained grasp.

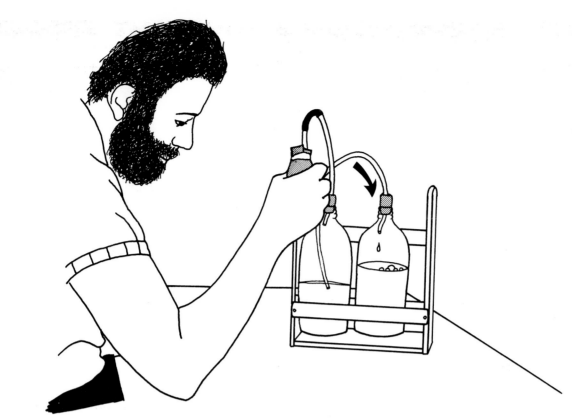

Gradation

	yes/no	How?
RESISTANCE	yes	alter elevation of second flask – if higher than the first flask, more pressure required and vice versa.
RANGE OF MOTION	yes	alter size of bulb.
CO-ORDINATION (gross/fine)	no	

Also used for:	How?
1 MCP flexion	to incorporate lumbricals, squeeze bulb using MCP flexion and fingers straight.
2 IP flexion	place bulb at MCPs and squeeze, using IP flexion.
3 Pinch	hold and squeeze bulb between thumb and distal end of each finger alternately; squeeze by pinching.

Comments

Fluid pumps are now commercially available.

TITLE ▮▮▮▮▮

Ping Pong Puff

MOVEMENT ▮▮▮

Grasp Strengthening

Category

Purposeful Activity, Moderate

Description

Patient grasps the rubber bulb in the palm of the hand and squeezes as hard as possible to move the ball up the track. Release and squeeze again. Record progress by noting the coloured section to which the patient is able to blow the ball.

Equipment

▶ ping pong ball;

▶ wooden track with air tube and bulb attached (*see Figure 1*).

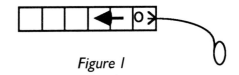

Figure 1

Skills required for activity as exercise
Action

Joints Used	Minimum Jt Range	Main Muscle Groups	Type of Contraction	Minimum Ms Grade
ACTIVE *Squeeze* MCPs/IPs thumb	$\sim\frac{1}{2}$ $\sim\frac{1}{2}$	flexors flexors	concentric concentric	3+ 3+
Release MCPs/IPs thumb	same same	extensors extensors	concentric concentric	3− 2
STATIC wrist				

Co-ordination

Gross Motor ■ none required except for trunk stability for sitting or standing; activity could also be done in lying position if necessary.

Fine Motor ■ controlled grasp/release.

Gradation

	yes/no	How?
RESISTANCE	yes	alter size and weight of ball used, eg. squash ball or polystyrene ball.
RANGE OF MOTION	yes	alter size of rubber bulb.
CO-ORDINATION (gross/fine)	no	

Also used for:	How?
1 MCP flexion	to incorporate lumbricals, squeeze bulb using MCP flexion and fingers straight.
2 IP flexion	place bulb at MCPs and squeeze using IP flexion.
3 Pinch	hold and squeeze bulb between thumb and distal end of each finger alternately; squeeze by pinching.

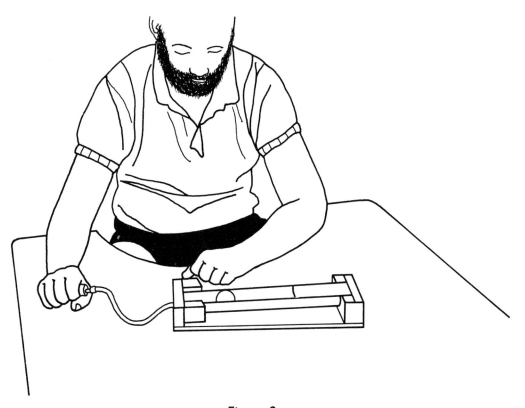

Figure 2

TITLE
Clothes-peg Sheep

MOVEMENT
Pinch Strengthening

Category

Purposeful Activity, Moderate

Description

Using a board (*see Figure 1*) with clothes-pegs as 'sheep', transpose the red and white clothes-pegs either by one move forward or by jumping forward over another clothes-peg – never go backwards. To complete the game, transpose colours again to original arrangement. Squeeze clothes-pegs between thumb and finger alternately.

Alternatively, just attach the clothes-pegs to a board (*see Figure 2*).

Equipment

▶ 'Sheep' board with clothes-peg pieces attached to thin pegs.

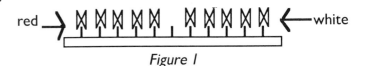

Figure 1

Skills required for activity as exercise
Action

Joints Used	Minimum Jt Range	Main Muscle Groups	Type of Contraction	Minimum Ms Grade
ACTIVE				
		Pinch		
MCPs/IPs	partial *	flexors	concentric	4
		intrinsics	concentric	4
thumb	a few degrees	flexors	concentric	4
		Release		
MCPs/IPs	as above	extensors	concentric	3–
thumb	as above	extensors	concentric	3

Co-ordination

Gross Motor ■ proximal control.

Fine Motor ■ acccurate targeting and placement;
■ controlled pinch/release.

Gradation

	yes/no	How?
RESISTANCE	yes	alter spring on clothes-peg; use removable pegs as sheep; use tweezers or tongs to move removable pegs.
RANGE OF MOTION	yes	alter size of clothes-pegs or pegs.
CO-ORDINATION (gross/fine)	no	

Also used for:	How?
1 IP flexion	same technique.
2 MCP flexion	to eliminate long flexors and use lumbricals, do with straight fingers.

Comments

* Range required depends on the size of the pegs. If someone has limited range but requires strengthening, clothes-pegs or pegs can be adapted at the top to decrease range requirements. Also, good thumb range can compensate for decreased finger range and vice versa – set clear goals and watch patient carefully to ensure goals are being achieved.

Can also be incorporated for use with any form of solitaire board.

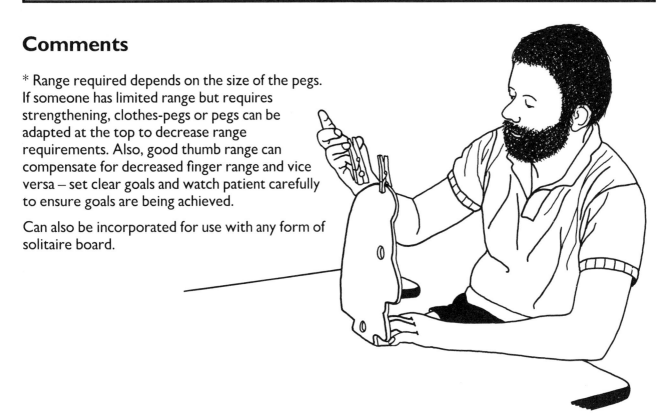

Figure 2

TITLE
Putty Pinch

MOVEMENT
Pinch Strengthening

Category

Therapeutic Exercise, Moderate

Equipment

▶ theraputty of varying densities (resistance).

Description

Patient sits at table with theraputty in front. Roll theraputty into a thick sausage shape and ask patient to pinch it between the thumb and each finger alternately for the length of the 'sausage'. Roll putty into 'sausage' again and repeat as many times as can be tolerated.

Skills required for activity as exercise
Action

Joints Used	Minimum Jt Range	Main Muscle Groups	Type of Contraction	Minimum Ms Grade
ACTIVE				
		Pinch		
MCPs/IPs	$\sim\frac{1}{3}$	flexors	concentric	4
		intrinsics	concentric	4
thumb	$\sim\frac{1}{3}$	flexors	concentric	4
		Release		
MCPs/IPs	as above	extensors	concentric	3—
thumb	as above	extensors	concentric	3—
STATIC wrist				

Co-ordination

Gross Motor ■ proximal control and sitting balance.

Fine Motor ■ controlled pinch/release;
■ does not require accurate fine control.

133

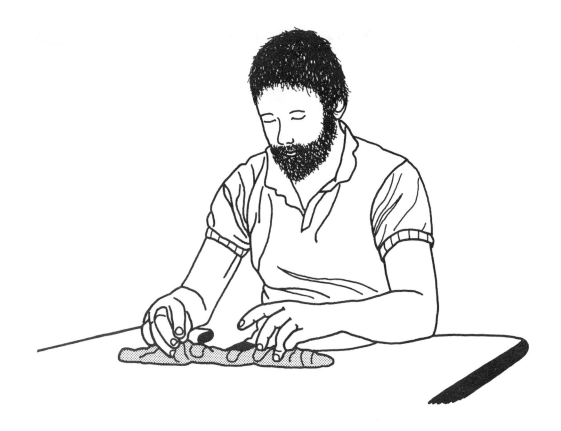

Gradation

	yes/no	How?
RESISTANCE	yes	alter density of theraputty used; pinch a variety of materials (eg. foam, paper, wet sponge).
RANGE OF MOTION	yes	alter thickness of 'sausage' squeezed; work within available range starting at $\sim\frac{1}{3}$.
CO-ORDINATION (gross/fine)	no	

Also used for:	How?
1 IP flexion	same technique as for pinch.
2 MCP flexion	pinch putty between thumb and straight fingers.
3 MCP abd/add.	pinch putty between fingers, keeping MCPs and IPs straight.

TITLE	MOVEMENT
Tweezer Bead Art	**Pinch Strengthening**

Category

Purposeful Activity, Moderate

Description

Patient sits at table with 'bead art' (board and beads) in front of them. Use tweezers, held between thumb and alternate finger tips, to pick up the beads and then place them in mounting board. To eliminate compensation at the MCPs, use a wooden 'butterfly' (*see Figure 1*) to block movement at the MCPs. Can put beads in board at random or in a selected pattern, as appropriate.

Equipment

▶ 'bead art' (commercially available), includes small coloured beads, designs and mounting board;

▶ tweezers of varying sizes and tensions;

▶ wooden 'butterflies' (*see Figure 2*).

Skills required for activity as exercise
Action

Joints Used	Minimum Jt Range	Main Muscle Groups	Type of Contraction	Minimum Ms Grade
ACTIVE *Close* IPs	$\sim\frac{1}{2}-\frac{3}{4}$	flexors intrinsics	concentric concentric	3+ 3+
thumb	$\sim\frac{1}{2}$	flexors	concentric	3+
Open IPs thumb	as above as above	extensors extensors	concentric concentric	3− 3−
STATIC MCPs wrist				

Co-ordination

Gross Motor ■ proximal control for accurate hand function.

Fine Motor ■ accurate targeting and placement;
■ controlled pinch/release;
■ good eye/hand co-ordination.

Gradation

	yes/no	How?
RESISTANCE	yes	place elastic bands around the end of the tweezers, alter tension of tweezers; can be done without tweezers, just using pinch to hold and move beads.
RANGE OF MOTION	yes	alter size of beads; alter size of tweezers.
CO-ORDINATION (gross/fine)	yes	alter size of beads and target – larger beads require less fine motor control.

Also used for:	How?
1 IP flex/ext.	same technique as for pinch strengthening; to ensure DIP flex. use 'butterfly' at mid-phalanx, for PIP flex. place 'butterfly' at proximal phalanx.
2 MCP flex/ext.	hold tweezers between thumb and straight fingers, flexing only at the MCPs.
3 MCP abd/add.	hold and squeeze tweezers between fingers, keeping MCPs straight.

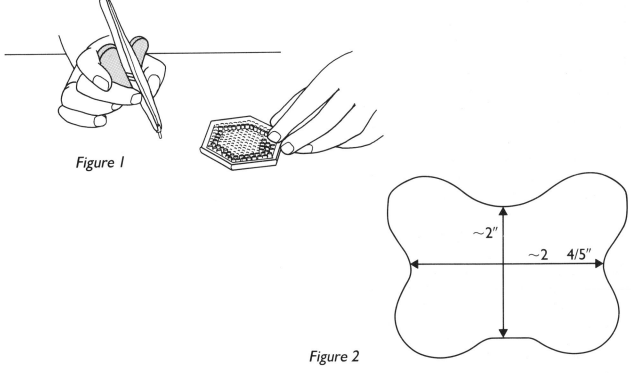

Figure 1

Figure 2

Size of butterfly can be altered according to hand size

~2"

~2 4/5"

Use of Computer Switches

There is a continuing need for innovative hand and arm exercising equipment in occupational therapy. New designs involving computer technology can provide an interesting and expansive tool which helps in the treatment of upper limb function. Some new devices are currently available while others are still at the developmental or prototype stages. Research in this area continues to assist occupational therapists in the development of more sophisticated, motivating and measurable activities.

The computer can offer exciting and motivating visual and auditory stimuli through software, and a multitude of specific exercises through varied input mechanisms. Tasks can be tailored to suit the needs of individual patient treatment. With the computer various parameters such as strength, range and speed can be altered as required, and therefore a graded activity provided. Also, those same parameters can be measured and graphed to provide a record of progress for the patient and therapist.

There is a large variety of input mechanisms that can be used, depending on the established therapeutic treatment goals. Some of the input devices available are: the touch screen, various keyboards, lightpens, joysticks, the mouse, a pressure and sensor bulb, and a large variety of switches including those operated by mercury, touch, pneumatics and mechanics. Exercise machines or special mechanical devices can also be adapted and attached to a micro-computer to control the desired software. The placement of and method in which the patient operates the input mechanism (eg. joystick, dual touch switch, FEPs) is of particular importance when using a computer game as a tool to achieve a specific physical exercise to improve dexterity, speed, range of movement or strength.

The software is important in that it provides the visual feedback as an incentive for the patient during the exercise. It also provides the patient and therapist with objective feedback on the patient's performance. The following components must be considered when selecting software for treatment: interest to the patient; level of challenge; age appropriateness; cognitive level required.

Computer software can also increase the number of ways in which control devices may be used. The range and/or speed of movement required can be specified and the level of difficulty, both cognitive and physical, can be altered. The strength required can only be adjusted by the means of hardware or input devices. Therefore the activities can be modified and measured through software and hardware to suit the specific requirements of the patient.

As in any other therapeutic activity, it is vital that the patient understand the treatment goals and find the chosen activity meaningful and motivating towards their rehabilitation goals. It is equally important that the therapist closely monitor the patient's performance of the chosen computer activity to ensure that the specific requirements, both physical and cognitive, are being adequately met and revised as necessary.

TITLE ██████

Computer Switch Protraction/ Retraction

MOVEMENT ██████

Shoulder Protraction/ Retraction

Category

Purposeful Activity, Light

Description

Patient sits with computer monitor in front of them. A joystick is mounted on table directly in front of patient's shoulder at shoulder height and arm's length away. The joystick is grasped with a palmar grasp and forearm in mid-position and elbow straight. It is activated by the forward and backward movement at the shoulder (that is, shoulder protraction/retraction). An appropriate

program (that is, according to age, cognitive level, and suitable to two-position joystick control) is inserted into the disk drive and patient controls it with the joystick.

Equipment

▶ computer including central processing unit, monitor, disk drive, and appropriate software;

▶ two-position, micro-switch joystick.

Skills required for activity as exercise
Action

Joints Used	Minimum Jt Range	Main Muscle Groups	Type of Contraction	Minimum Ms Grade
ACTIVE *Forward* shoulder	$\sim\frac{1}{2}$ range prot/retr.	protractors	concentric	3+
Pull Back shoulder	as above	retractors	concentric	3+
STATIC shoulder at $\sim70°–90°$ elbow — fully extended wrist hand — grasp				

Co-ordination

Gross Motor ■ control at shoulder, co-ordination between protractors and retractors;

■ can be done as an active assisted, bilateral activity by grasping the joystick with clasped hands.

Fine Motor ■ sustained palmar grasp (this can be eliminated by attaching a strap or 'C-Clip' to joystick; patient's hand is then supported by that).

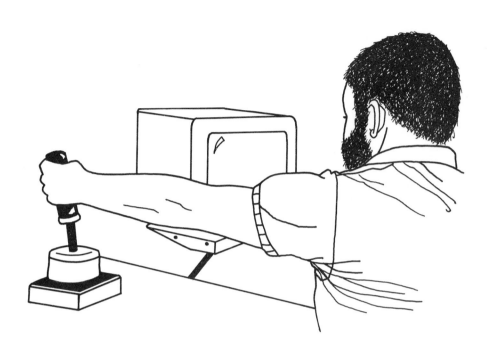

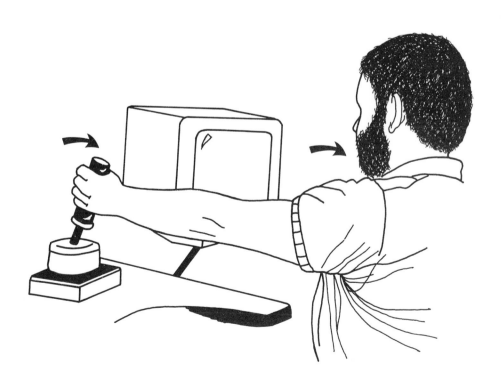

Gradation

	yes/no	How?
RESISTANCE	yes	it is possible with some switches to alter the tension (check with an engineer); add wrist cuffs to patient.
RANGE OF MOTION	yes	set joystick to patient's maximum range by adding stop; then alter program to accommodate switch change (see engineer).
CO-ORDINATION (gross/fine)	yes	make this either a unilateral or active assisted bilateral activity.

Also used for:	How?
1 elbow flex/ext.	elbow is not kept straight, rather the joystick is controlled by using elbow flexion and extension alternately.
2 wrist flex/ext.	joystick is controlled by wrist flexion and extension alternately.

Comments

The computer can provide excellent motivation if used carefully and only with appropriate programs. For switch design and adaptations, seek the assistance of your local engineer.

TITLE ▮▮▮▮▮▮▮▮
Computerised FEPS

MOVEMENT ▮▮▮▮▮
Pronation/ Supination

Category

Purposeful Activity, Light

Description

Patient sits in front of micro-computer with FEPS set up on side to be exercised. The appropriate handle is selected and attached to the FEPS unit. The appropriate computer game is selected, patient instructed as to use of the FEPS and the game. Patient grasps handle and controls game by moving the handle with pronation/supination alternately. Keep elbow flexed to 90° and close to side at all times.

Equipment

▶ micro-computer including central processing unit, monitor, disk drive;

▶ FEPS attachment with transducers*, FEPS handle attachments;

▶ compatible and appropriate software.

Skills required for activity as exercise
Action

Joints Used	Minimum Jt Range	Main Muscle Groups	Type of Contraction	Minimum Ms Grade
ACTIVE rad/ul. joints	~$\frac{1}{2}$	pronators supinators	conc/ecc. (vv) ecc/conc. (vv)	3 3
STATIC elbow — flexed to 90° hand — gross grasp wrist — in neutral				

Co-ordination

Gross Motor ■ control at elbow and radial/ulnar joints;
■ amount of co-ordination and accuracy required depends on computer game used; can be graded.

Fine Motor ■ sustained gross grasp.

Gradation

	yes/no	How?
RESISTANCE	no **	
RANGE OF MOTION	yes	can programme computer for maximum range available.
CO-ORDINATION (gross/fine)	yes	alter program used (eg. vary speed, co-ordination and accuracy requirements).

Also used for:	How?
1 wrist flex/ext.	patient sits sideways to the computer and uses wrist flex/ext. alternately to operate the FEPS control.
2 IP extension	use large span grip; patient opens hand to grasp the handle, using maximum IP range; operate the FEPS control by twisting the span grip control.

Comments

* This equipment is not yet commercially available and is still in the research phase. However, it has been tested successfully in clinical settings and further research continues. The idea is not copy-righted!

** To date resistance cannot be altered, so that this is an exercise for range of motion, but not for strengthening. However, future developments should incorporate a resistance factor.

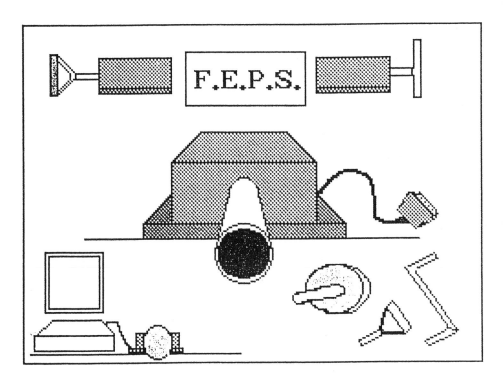

TITLE
Mercury Switch with Computer

MOVEMENT
Pronation/ Supination

Category

Purposeful Activity, Light

Description

Patient sits with arm at side, elbow bent to 90°, and forearm in mid-position. Attach the mercury switch to a wrist band and place on wrist, at resting position in neutral. Play game that can be controlled with the dual mercury switch, using pronation and supination to activate. Keep elbow in at side.

Equipment

▶ micro-computer including central processing unit, monitor, disk drive;

▶ mercury activation switch attached by velcro to wrist band;

▶ compatible and appropriate software.

Skills required for activity as exercise
Action

Joints Used	Minimum Jt Range	Main Muscle Groups	Type of Contraction	Minimum Ms Grade
ACTIVE rad/ul. joints.	$\sim\frac{1}{4}$	supinators pronators	conc/ecc. (vv) ecc/conc. (vv)	3 3
STATIC elbow at $\sim$90°				

Co-ordination

Gross Motor ■ co-ordination between pronators and supinators;
■ ability to react to action on computer screen.

Fine Motor ■ none.

Gradation

	yes/no	How?
RESISTANCE	yes	add weighted wrist cuffs to increase resistance.
RANGE OF MOTION	yes	programme computer to operate within minimum and maximum range available.
CO-ORDINATION (gross/fine)	yes	alter programme speed and complexity.

Also used for:	How?
shoulder rotation	place switch on wrist, keep elbow straight and shoulder flexed to 90°; activate switch by using shoulder internal and external rotation alternately.

Comments

Computers can be excellent motivators if an appropriate game is selected. Be sure to select appropriate software, considering age, cognitive level, and compatibility with switch.

TITLE

Computer Switch Elevation/Depression

MOVEMENT

Shoulder Elevation/Depression

Category

Purposeful Activity, Light

Equipment

▶ computer including central processing unit, monitor, disk drive;

▶ appropriate software, that is, in consideration of age and cognitive level of patient, and software that can be controlled with two switches;

▶ two touch or mechanical switches with attachment hardware.

Description

Patient sits in front of the computer. A computer switch (either touch sensitive or mechanical) is mounted on the chair back just over the top of the shoulder, and another mounted just below the elbow, which is flexed to 90° (*see Figure 1*). The switches are activated by shoulder elevation and depression alternately. An appropriate computer program is inserted into the disk drive and then controlled by the two shoulder switches.

Skills required for activity as exercise
Action

Joints Used	Minimum Jt Range	Main Muscle Groups	Type of Contraction	Minimum Ms Grade
ACTIVE *Top Switch* shoulder *Elbow Switch* shoulder	~$\frac{1}{2}$ elev. full depression	elevators depressors	concentric concentric	3+ 2 (gravity assists)
STATIC elbow — flexed to 90°				

Co-ordination

Gross Motor ■ control at the shoulder, with co-ordination between shoulder elevators and depressors;
■ speed and accuracy required depends on the computer used.

Fine Motor ■ none.

Gradation

	yes/no	How?
RESISTANCE	yes	can put weights (eg. sand bags) over shoulder.
RANGE OF MOTION	yes	alter placement of switches (that is, place to achieve maximum range available).
CO-ORDINATION (gross/fine)	yes	depends on the computer program used.

Also used for:	How?
any desired movement	place switches within maximum range of any movement; watch carefully for compensatory movements.

Comment

Ensure that patient fully understands the computer game or activity and that it is age and cognitively appropriate before use.

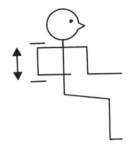

Index

Elbow Flexion/Extension — 61

Darts	80
Guillotining	37
Kneading	10
Knights*	62
Magic Squares	20
Pyramids	50
Rolling Pastry	16
Sanding	34
Sheep	74
Shove Board*	64
Skateboard	26
Spot Board	28
Suspended Ball Activity	59
Tug O'War I	18

Finger Abduction/Adduction — 105

Coin Travel*	106
Interossei Box*	108
Interossei Sheep*	110
Tug O'War II*	112

Grasp Strengthening — 127

Fluid Pump*	127
Ping Pong Puff*	129
Sponge Ball Squeeze	99

IP Flexion/Extension — 115

Bandage Roll	90
Beads*	118
Clothes-Peg Sheep	131
Elastics*	120
Finger Extension Game	93
Fluid Pump	127
Interossei Sheep	110
Nuts and Bolts*	116
Pin Solitaire*	125
Ping Pong Puff	129
Putty Pancake*	123
Sponge Ball Squeeze	99
Tong Solitaire	103
T-Shaped Solitaire	101

MCP Flexion/Extension — 89

Bandage Roll*	90
Beads	118
Clothes-Peg Sheep	131
Elastics	120
Finger Extension Game*	93
Finger Ladder	46
Fluid Pump	127
Lumbrical Box Game*	95
Lumbrical Sanding*	97
Pin Solitaire	125
Ping Pong Puff	129
Putty Pancake	123
Ski Jump	84
Sponge Ball Squeeze*	99
Tong Solitaire*	103
T-Shaped Solitaire*	101

Pinch Strengthening — 131

Beads	118
Clothes-peg Sheep*	131
Fluid Pump	127
Interossei Sheep	110
Nuts and Bolts	116
Pin Solitaire	125
Ping Pong Puff	129
Putty Pinch*	133
Sponge Ball Squeeze	99
Tong Solitaire	103
Tweezer Bead Art*	135

Forearm Pronation/Supination — 67

Computerised FEPS*	141
Dowel: pronation/supination*	68
Dowel: shoulder rotation	54
Mercury Switch with Computer*	143
Pyramids	50
Sheep*	74
Stick Printing	56
Table Football*	77
Threaded Solitaire I*	72
Wire Maze*	70

Shoulder Abduction/Adduction 43

Braintease*	44
Bricks	32
Dowel: shoulder abduction/adduction*	48
Finger Ladder*	46
Guillotining	37
Knights	62
Pyramids*	50
Sanding	34
Stick Printing	56

Shoulder Depression/Elevation 9

Computer Switch Elevation/Depression	145
Kneading*	10
Maze Game*	12

Shoulder Extension/Flexion 31

Braintease	44
Bricks*	32
Chopping*	40
Finger Ladder	46
Guillotining*	37
Knights	62
Magic Squares	20
Pyramids	50
Rolling Pastry	16
Sanding*	34
Sheep	74
Stick Printing	56
Tug O' War I	18

Shoulder Horizontal Abduction/Adduction 23

Chopping	40
Dowel: horizontal abduction/adduction*	24
Sanding	34
Shove Board	64
Skateboard*	26
Spot Board*	28
Suspended Ball Activity	59

Shoulder Protraction/Retraction 15

Computer Switch Protraction/Retraction*	138
Knights	62
Magic Squares*	20
Rolling Pastry*	16
Skateboard	26
Suspended Ball Activity	59
Tug O' War I*	18

Shoulder Rotation 53

Dowel: pronation/supination	68
Dowel: shoulder rotation*	54
Pyramids	50
Sheep	74
Stick Printing*	56
Suspended Ball Activity*	59
Threaded Solitaire I	72
Wire Maze	70

Tenodesis Training

Knights	62
Pyramids	50
Ski Jump	84

Wrist Flexion/Extension 79

Darts*	80
Finger Extension Game	93
Post Box*	82
Sanding	34
Ski Jump*	84
Spot Board	28
Stick Printing	56
Threaded Solitaire II*	86
Wire Maze	70

* The asterisk shows that the activity is described under this section.